Recent Advances in the Health Benefits of Tea

Edited by Christophe Hano and Samantha Drouet

Published in London, United Kingdom

Recent Advances in the Health Benefits of Tea
http://dx.doi.org/10.5772/intechopen.102174
Edited by Christophe Hano and Samantha Drouet

Contributors
Bowen Liu, Jun Zhang, Guanben Du, Xiaojian Zhou, Shuduan Deng, Graham Johnston, Tina Hinton, Kong M. Li, Vincent Viengkhou, Sandra Kindaro, Herbert F. Jelinek, Sin Yoo Kam, Slade Matthews, Sabila Nelson, Abdulloh Machin, Shafira Putri Widiawan, Neil Shay, Alexandra Becraft, Ruhul Amin, Biplab Kumar Dey, Nasreddine El Omari, Abdelhakim Bouyahya, Samantha Drouet, Javad Sharifi-Rad, Christophe F.E. Hano

First published in London, United Kingdom, 2023 by IntechOpen
IntechOpen is the global imprint of INTECHOPEN LIMITED, registered in England and Wales, registration number: 11086078, 5 Princes Gate Court, London, SW7 2QJ, United Kingdom

British Library Cataloguing-in-Publication Data
A catalogue record for this book is available from the British Library

Additional hard and PDF copies can be obtained from orders@intechopen.com

Recent Advances in the Health Benefits of Tea
Edited by Christophe Hano and Samantha Drouet
p. cm.
Print ISBN 978-1-80355-663-5
Online ISBN 978-1-80355-664-2
eBook (PDF) ISBN 978-1-80355-665-9

Meet the editors

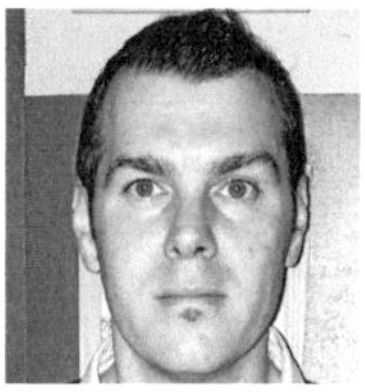

Dr. Christophe Hano is a phytochemist and an assistant professor at the University of Orléans, France. His research interests include plant-specialized metabolism and plant biotechnology for nutraceutical, medicinal, and cosmeceutical applications. He has published more than 250 scientific papers, reviews, and book chapters in internationally renowned journals, as well as edited one book and many journal issues.

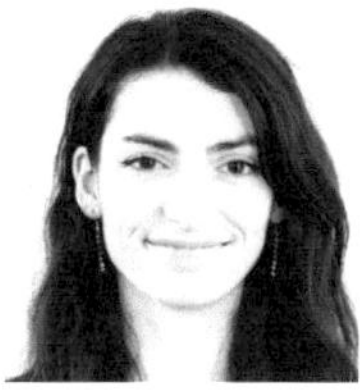

Dr. Samantha Drouet is a plant biochemist. Her main interest is in the valorization of plant secondary metabolites with pharmaceutical, nutraceutical or cosmeceutical interest. She has a strong background in green extraction methodologies and biotechnologies. She is the author of more than 50 scientific papers, reviews and book chapters for internationally renowned journals and publishers.

Contents

Preface

Plants have always offered an inexhaustible source of active compounds for human health and well-being. Plants and their preparations are used in various traditional medicines for the treatment, prevention, and diagnosis of disease. Plants and traditional remedies derived from them continue to be an important source of inspiration for so-called contemporary medicine, which can aid in the (re)discovery of new treatments, as evidenced by the success of the antimalarial artemisinin. The discovery of several important bioactive chemicals in plants used in traditional Chinese, Indian, Japanese, Thai, Korean, African, American, and European medicines shows that artemisinin is not an isolated example.

Tea is one of the most popular beverages in the world, and the second most consumed after water. Based on evidence from cellular, animal, epidemiological, and clinical studies, tea consumption has been linked to several health benefits, including cancer chemoprevention, chronic inflammation, heart and liver diseases, diabetes, and neurodegenerative disorders. Even though not all health advantages have been consistently established, several clinical trial findings have provided tangible data proving green tea's health benefits, including cancer-protective effects. The effects of tea processing and storage, as well as additives, on the characteristics and health activity of tea have also been investigated.

The aim of the present book, *Recent Advances in the Health Benefits of Tea*, is to combine review and research chapters to elucidate tea's health benefits, including the molecular targets, biological processes, and mechanisms of action involved.

Dr. Christophe Hano and Dr. Samantha Drouet
Department of Biochemistry,
University of Orléans,
Orléans, France

Chapter 1

Green Tea and Its Numerous Health Benefits

Ruhul Amin, Biplab Kumar Dey, Nasreddine El Omari, Abdelhakim Bouyahya, Samantha Drouet, Christophe Hano and Javad Sharifi-Rad

Abstract

Green tea is one of the most popular antioxidant drinks in the world. To make green tea, you must first remove the leaves from *Camellia sinensis*. A form of tea made from unoxidized green leaves from a tea plantation is called green tea. Several other studies have been undertaken over the past year to evaluate whether consuming green tea and extracts has any health benefits. In order to get the health benefits of green tea, the nutrients in the tea must be absorbed. Green tea's flavonoids and caffeine, which serve to accelerate the elimination of metabolites, contribute to the antioxidant function of green tea. Cancer, heart disease, and aging appear to be the main diseases to be reduced or prevented by these antioxidants. The pharmaceutical and culinary industries can use green tea due to its high potency and lack of adverse effects. Green tea is touted as a natural remedy for a wide range of health issues. Through this, we can better understand the immediate benefits of green tea. Prescription green tea components are discussed along with their antioxidant, anticancer, and antiviral actions in relation to the treatment of cardiovascular diseases (CVD).

Keywords: green tea, antioxidant, cardiovascular diseases, health benefits

1. Introduction

The *Camellia Sinensis* plant, from which tea is produced, is cultivated in more than 30 countries throughout the globe [1, 2]. White tea, green tea, black tea, and oolong tea are the four varieties of tea produced [3, 4]. This type of tea is made from the same plant, *C. Sinensis*, as the previous varieties. White tea undergoes the least processing, followed by green tea, which are both unfermented, oolong tea, which is partially fermented, and black tea, which is fermented, all of which undergo an oxidation process before being consumed [5]. Compare to other teas, green tea is among the least oxidized. Green tea is available in many forms, such as tea bags. Loose-leaf, instant power, and supplement sold in capsule form. It is made from unfermented leaves with minimal processing and contains catechin (80–90%) and flavanols (<10%) [6]. It provides a high concentration of antioxidants called polyphenols. Currently, green tea is mostly consumed in China, Japan, and Korea. It is responsible for improving blood circulation, lowering cholesterol levels, preventing a variety of cardiovascular problems, and protecting against the harmful effects of a high-fat diet [7, 8]. Worldwide, black tea accounts for around 78% of total consumption, and green tea accounts for approximately 20% [9, 10]. Green tea can bring relaxation and a calm feeling to its lovers, unlike soft drinks or liquors.

2. Research methodology

Data for this research was sourced from Pub Med, Science Direct, Google Scholar, the World Wide Web of Science, and Cochrane review. We used a variety of keywords, including "Green Tea," "Tea AND health Benefits," "herb," "herbal Medicines," and "Green Tea AND Cancer" to search these databases.

3. Results and discussion

3.1 History

The history of tea drinking started in 2737 BC. AD, according to Chinese tradition, when Emperor Shen Nong, a skilled ruler and scientific trained, discovered tea by mistake [11, 12]. *Camellia* species have spread from Nepal to Taiwan. Japan in East Asia has more than 90 species, tea is the most distributed [13, 14].

Green tea is very popular in East Asia (especially in China and Japan), while black tea is in the West. The use of tea leaves probably began in southwestern China over 3000 years ago. It was initially used only for chewing and drinking, much like using coffee for the first time [15]. The origin of the tea plantation was estimated by Sealy [16] around the Chinese Yunnan district, but it is not confirmed. Wild form of the Assamica variety of *C. Sinensis* was discovered in India in 1835, then in Thailand and Burma [17, 18].

3.2 Green tea composition

The chemical composition of green tea differs from climatic, seasonal, horticultural, and foliar synthesis [19]. The most important components of green tea are polyphenols. The catechins make up 80–90% of the flavonoids and about 40% of the water solids in green tea [20]. Green tea contains more catechins than other forms of tea. It is mainly due to post-harvest processing. The four main catechins contained in green tea are (−)-epicatechin (EC), (−)-epigallocatechin (ECG), (−)-epicatechin 3-gallate (ECG), and (−)-epigallocatechin gallate (EGCG) [21, 22] (**Figure 1**). EGCG, having the high concentration, has been widely studied for its health benefits. It contains (~60%), followed by EGC (~20%), ECG (~14%), and EC (~6%) (**Figure 2**). As mentioned above, the amount of catechins in any specific green tea beverage can vary greatly. At the same time, the standardized extract is available for use in addition [23].

3.3 Medicinal value of green tea

3.3.1 Antioxidant properties

Different compounds found in green tea showed significant *in vitro* and *in vivo* antioxidant effects. Indeed, ECGC-specific green tea originating from catechin is a

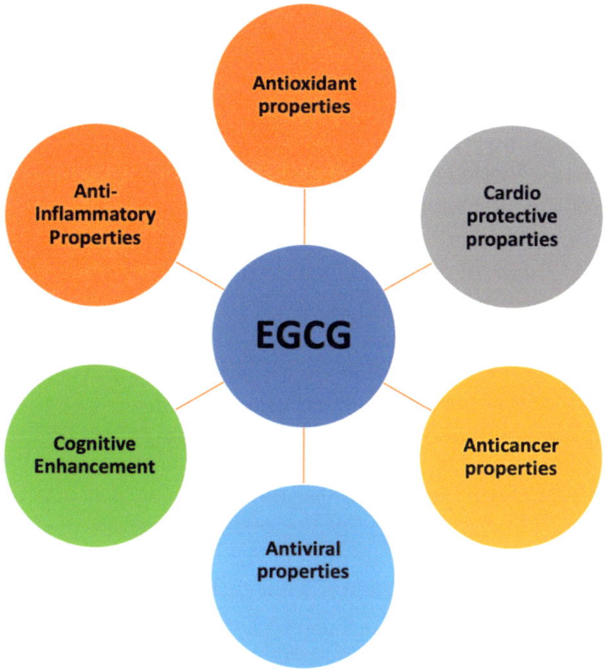

Figure 1.
Different benefits of green tea.

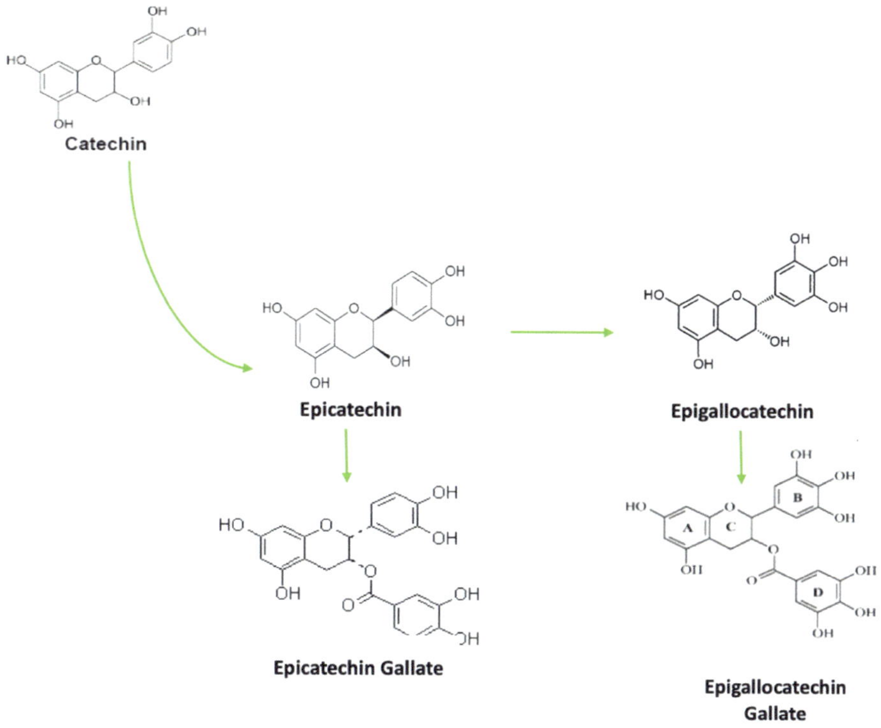

Figure 2.
Different forms of catechins.

potent antioxidant capable of inhibiting the growth of cancer cells [24]. Green tea can boost humoral and cell-mediated immunity and reduce the risk of cancer and cardiovascular diseases. ECGC is responsible for much of the chemopreventive properties of green tea against cancer [25]. It is suggested to induce apoptosis and promote the arrest of cell growth by alternating expression of cellular regulatory proteins [25]. As already mentioned, green tea contains a large amount of antioxidants called polyphenols. There is ample evidence supporting the ability of green tea flavonoids to prevent tumors by suppressing free radical production [26–28]. These antioxidants can slow or inhibit the development of cancer and heart disease, promote immune function, and delay the aging process (**Figure 1**) [29–32].

3.3.2 Cardioprotective diseases protection

Cardiovascular diseases (CVD) are unpredictable problems that include various variables. Associated risk factors include irritation, oxidative pressure, platelet total, and lipid digestion. In recent years, many studies have focused on the possibility of using green tea against CVD [33, 34]. Smoke-related heart disease is associated with several risk factors. They are most common in the western world, likely due to the lifestyle in this part of the world, which involves a diet high in saturated fats and low physical activities [35, 36].

It has been reported that people who drink at least 3 cups of green tea per day have a 2% lower risk of stroke compared to those who drink less than one cup a day [37]. Regular consumption of green tea tends to reduce the risk of high blood pressure.

One of the causes of high blood pressure is the lack of arterial elasticity. Over time, this elasticity is lost and one of the causes of arterial constriction is thromboxane. The source of hypertension is an enzyme called angiotensin-converting enzymes (ACE), which is secreted by the kidney. Green tea has been reported to inhibit the activity of this enzyme, which significantly lowers blood pressure [30, 38].

3.3.3 Anticancer properties

A variety of studies based on people's dietary habits have confirmed the anticancer effect of green tea [39, 40]. For example, the cancer incidence rate tends to be low in countries like Japan, where green tea is regularly consumed. One of the benefits of green tea is that carcinogenesis in the digestive tract is believed to be inhibited by the action of ECGC [41, 42].

Colorectal cancer may be prevented or delayed by adopting a healthy diet and lifestyle. Obesity increases the risk of developing abdominal cancer, especially if the obesity is visceral and results from an unhealthy lifestyle that lasts for a long time [43]. Colorectal cancer may be less likely to occur if EGCG consumption inhibits tumor growth factors. Apoptosis, or programmed cell death, caused by EGCG may also be a way to kill cancer cells. Obesity-related carcinogenesis may be reduced by increasing insulin and leptin tissue sensitivity and decreasing blood lipid levels. Recurrent adenomas, which in the majority of cases can progress to colorectal cancer, may be prevented by taking green tea extract supplements [44]. According to numerous studies, EGCG supplementation can reduce the risk of cancer in the gallbladder and bile ducts [45, 46].

Treatment, as well as prevention against cancer, may involve the use of catechins [47]. The anti-cancer activities of vitamin C have been linked to its antioxidant abilities [48, 49].

3.3.4 Antiviral properties

Patients suffering from infectious disorders, including COVID-19, may benefit from green tea's immunomodulatory and antiviral characteristics [50, 51]. There are several types of research on the antiviral activities of green tea, but most of them are based on traditional accounts [8, 10, 32, 52, 53]. Despite the fact that green tea has a special composition and ratio of bioactive components, the mechanism of action and distinctive features of green tea remain a mystery. It is still possible that matcha green tea has antiviral properties (by inactivating SARS-CoV-2), as proven by Ohgitani et al. in one of the few trials, but additional research is required [54]. Chemicals found in green tea that

Activities	Green tea Active compounds	Mechanisms of Action	References
Cardio-protective properties	EGCG	Inhibited stress-induced protein kinase activation and other inflammation-inducing signaling pathways	[55, 56]
	Rutin	Induced vascular support	[57]
Anticancer properties	Catechins	Inhibited tumor growth factors Induced cancer cell apoptosis	[44, 47]
	Vitamin C	Prevented and treated cancer	[48, 49]
	Phenolic acids	Inhibited cancer cell development Avoided metastases	[52]
	EGCG	Induced antioxidant effects Reduced inflammatory mechanisms causing hyperproliferation and onset of carcinogenesis Increased insulin and leptin sensitivity Decreased lipid levels	[44, 45, 47, 53]
Antiviral properties	Catechins	Inhibited SARS-Cov-2 primary proteases Disrupted viral replication cycle Inhibited HCV replication	[58–61]
	EGCG	Inhibited SARS-CoV-2 main protease and SARS-CoV-2-like protease 3C	[54, 59, 62–67]
	Quercetin	Inhibited SARS-Cov replication by protease inhibitors	[68]
	Catechins and quercetin	Inhibited structural proteins and primary protease of COVID-19	[50]
Anti-inflammatory properties	EGCG	Reduced inflammation by neutralizing oxidative stress	[69, 70]
Cognitive enhancement properties	Caffeine	Inhibited the aging process of the brain by reversing oxidative processes, and reducing neuroinflammation reduced cognitive loss likelihood	[71–74]
Preventive properties against neurodegenerative diseases	EGCG	Inhibited ROS formation Increased insulin sensitivity Reduced brain amyloid buildup	[75–77]

Table 1.
Summary of studies on green tea's health benefits.

have been researched for their putative properties and possible modes of action are listed in **Table 1**.

3.4 Anti-inflammatory properties

Many disorders are accompanied by an inflammatory response. Chemicals that encourage the production of reactive oxygen species (ROS), which may cause cell damage and long-term dysfunction throughout the body, can induce inflammation and cell damage. Anti-inflammatory and antioxidant compounds have the primary function of scavenging ROS and inhibiting inflammatory signaling [78].

EGCG, the main bioactive component of green tea, may reduce inflammation-related side effects, such as lung damage and dysfunction, after major heart surgery, including cardiopulmonary bypass [79, 80]. Gallstone development is less likely when the inflammatory state is controlled by this molecule. Several genes regulate high blood pressure, and inflammation and vascular remodeling are thought to play a role in its development [70, 81]. The consumption of green tea drinks containing high levels of bioactive components that regulate inflammatory processes has been shown to reduce the risk of developing hepatitis.

3.4.1 Cognitive enhancement and neurodegenerative disease prevention

Drinking green tea has been shown to improve mental clarity and cognitive functioning. EGCG is the key ingredient for these health benefits [76]. Age-related cognitive declines can be influenced by several variables, including lifestyle [82]. Caffeine consumption, especially in older women, appears to have a protective effect against cognitive deterioration [73]. Caffeine's ability to reverse oxidative processes and reduce neuroinflammation may help keep the brain healthy as we age [74]. Memory loss may be caused by oxidative stress, which may cause neuronal damage. As a potent anti-inflammatory agent, caffeine administration may help to keep this condition at bay [71]. Caffeine's protective effects on the nervous system and its ability to delay the onset of neurodegenerative illnesses are directly related to its ability to reduce amyloid- deposits in the brain [72]. Lipopolysaccharide (LPS)-induced systemic inflammation plays an important role in neurodegenerative disorders. EGCG inhibits LPS-induced reactive nitrogen species (RNS) production, showing that it is a potent and effective neuroprotective treatment for neurological diseases caused by inflammation [77]. Consumption of EGCG improves cognitive performance, insulin sensitivity, and brain amyloid- formation; reduces neuroinflammation; and prevents neuropathologies associated with neurodegenerative disorders, such as Alzheimer's disease.

4. Future prospects

Green tea has a unique blend of health benefits due to its bioactive components shown in **Table 1**. As a result, green tea has higher concentrations of phenolic acids, quercetin, rutin, theanine, and chlorophyll than other varieties. It is an entirely new product that cannot be compared to any other green tea on the market today. The administration of its infusions and extracts may be effective in the prevention of free radicals and inflammatory disorders, as well as premature aging. The convenience of powdered green tea makes it an excellent meal supplement. Green tea's health benefits have not been properly studied. Several elements of its function, including its interactions with the gut microbiota and its impact on infectious diseases, warrant further study in this area. More research will be needed to prove the health benefits of green tea, including further examination of green tea's chemical composition, and further *in vitro* and *in vivo* studies. Additional randomized clinical trials (RCT) research is also required. Moreover, pharmacodynamic and pharmacokinetic aspects of identified compounds should be investigated to validate their actions and well as their bioavailability. On the other hand, toxicological investigations of green tea main compounds should be carried out with different doses and several periods to validate their safety.

5. Conclusion

Green tea antioxidants are attracting increasing attention due to their potential for application in preventive medicine and in the food industry, as well as their pharmacological effectiveness and lack of adverse effects. Growing awareness of antioxidant phytoconstituents and their use in diet and daily use may provide the human body with potential support to combat these diseases. Green tea is becoming a natural remedy for a wide range of health issues. With the latest technological advancements, the different abilities of green tea have been explored. Recent use of green tea in nanotechnology has indicated promising evidence for its bioavailability using lipid nanocapsules and liposome encapsulation to deliver EGCG. These results are encouraging. Many of these properties of green tea have been discovered through numerous preclinical studies, and there is still a lack of human clinical evidence for them. Thus for green tea to be used as a safe and effective medicine, there is an urgent need to test the efficacy, health, and translation guidelines.

Abbreviations

ACE	Angiotensin-Converting Enzymes
CVD	Cardiovascular Diseases
EC	(−)-Epicatechin
ECG	(−)-Epicatechin 3-Gallate
EGC	Epigallocatechin
EGCG	(−)-Epigallocatechin Gallate
LPS	Lipopolysaccharide
RNS	Reactive Nitrogen Species
ROS	Reactive Oxygen Species

Author details

Ruhul Amin[1], Biplab Kumar Dey[1], Nasreddine El Omari[2], Abdelhakim Bouyahya[3*], Samantha Drouet[4], Christophe Hano[4] and Javad Sharifi-Rad[5*]

1 Faculty of Pharmaceutical Science, Assam Down Town University, Guwahati, Assam, India

2 Faculty of Medicine and Pharmacy, Laboratory of Histology, Embryology, and Cytogenetic, Mohammed V University in Rabat, Morocco

3 Faculty of Sciences, Laboratory of Human Pathologies Biology, Department of Biology, Mohammed V University, Rabat, Morocco

4 Laboratoire de Biologie Des Ligneux Et Des Grandes Cultures (LBLGC), INRA USC1328 Université d'Orléans, France

5 Facultad de Medicina, Universidad del Azuay, Cuenca, Ecuador

*Address all correspondence to: boyahyaa-90@hotmail.fr; hano@univ-orleans.fr and javad.sharifirad@gmail.com

References

[1] Dias T. White tea (Camellia sinensis (L.)): An-tioxidant properties and beneficial health effects. International Journal of Food Science and Nutritional Diet. 2013;**2**(2):19-26

[2] Namita P, Mukesh R, Vijay KJ. Camellia sinensis (green tea): A review. Global Journal of Pharmacology. 2012;**6**(2):52-59

[3] Hilal Y, Engelhardt U. Characterisation of white tea–comparison to green and black tea. Journal für Verbraucherschutz und Lebensmittelsicherheit. 2007;**2**(4):414-421

[4] Kuo K-L, Weng M-S, Chiang C-T, Tsai Y-J, Lin-Shiau S-Y, Lin J-K. Comparative studies on the hypolipidemic and growth suppressive effects of oolong, black, pu-erh, and green tea leaves in rats. Journal of Agricultural and Food Chemistry. 2005;**53**(2):480-489

[5] Carloni P, Tiano L, Padella L, Bacchetti T, Customu C, Kay A, et al. Antioxidant activity of white, green and black tea obtained from the same tea cultivar. Food Research International. 2013;**53**(2):900-908

[6] Payne MJ, Hurst WJ, Miller KB, Rank C, Stuart DA. Impact of fermentation, drying, roasting, and Dutch processing on epicatechin and catechin content of cacao beans and cocoa ingredients. Journal of Agricultural and Food Chemistry. 2010;**58**(19):10518-10527

[7] Sumpio BE, Cordova AC, Berke-Schlessel DW, Qin F, Chen QH. Green tea, the "Asian paradox," and cardiovascular disease. Journal of the American College of Surgeons. 2006;**202**(5):813-825

[8] Wolfram S. Effects of green tea and EGCG on cardiovascular and metabolic health. Journal of the American College of Nutrition. 2007;**26**(4):373S-388S

[9] Sun C-L, Yuan J-M, Koh W-P, Yu MC. Green tea, black tea and breast cancer risk: A meta-analysis of epidemiological studies. Carcinogenesis. 2006;**27**(7):1310-1315

[10] Wang Z-M, Zhou B, Wang Y-S, Gong Q-Y, Wang Q-M, Yan J-J, et al. Black and green tea consumption and the risk of coronary artery disease: A meta-analysis. The American Journal of Clinical Nutrition. 2011;**93**(3):506-515

[11] Campbell D. The Tea Book. Pelican Publishing; 1995

[12] Ukers WH. All About Tea. Vol. 1. Tea and Coffee Trade Journal Company; 1935

[13] Long C-L, Li H, Ouyang Z, Yang X, Li Q, Trangmar B. Strategies for agrobiodiversity conservation and promotion: A case from Yunnan, China. Biodiversity & Conservation. 2003;**12**(6):1145-1156

[14] Shrivastava RR, Pateriya P, Singh M. Green tea-a short review. International Journal of Indigenous Herbs and Drugs. 2018;**3**(2):12-21

[15] Mair VH, Hoh E. The True History of Tea. Thames & Hudson; 2012

[16] Sealy JR. A Revision of the Genus Camellia. London: Royal Horticultural Society; 1958

[17] Hall N. The Tea Industry. Elsevier; 2000

[18] Martin LC. A History of Tea: The Life and Times of the World's Favorite Beverage. Tuttle Publishing; 2018

[19] Lin Y-L, Juan I-M, Chen Y-L, Liang Y-C, Lin J-K. Composition of polyphenols in fresh tea leaves and associations of their oxygen-radical-absorbing capacity with antiproliferative actions in fibroblast cells. Journal of Agricultural and Food Chemistry. 1996;**44**(6):1387-1394

[20] Sutherland BA, Rahman RM, Appleton I. Mechanisms of action of green tea catechins, with a focus on ischemia-induced neurodegeneration. The Journal of Nutritional Biochemistry. 2006;**17**(5):291-306

[21] Balentine DA, Wiseman SA, Bouwens LC. The chemistry of tea flavonoids. Critical Reviews in Food Science & Nutrition. 1997;**37**(8):693-704

[22] Park HS, Lee HJ, Shin MH, Lee K-W, Lee H, Kim Y-S, et al. Effects of cosolvents on the decaffeination of green tea by supercritical carbon dioxide. Food Chemistry. 2007;**105**(3):1011-1017

[23] Bettuzzi S, Brausi M, Rizzi F, Castagnetti G, Peracchia G, Corti A. Chemoprevention of human prostate cancer by oral administration of green tea catechins in volunteers with high-grade prostate intraepithelial neoplasia: A preliminary report from a one-year proof-of-principle study. Cancer Research. 2006;**66**(2):1234-1240

[24] Du G-J, Zhang Z, Wen X-D, Yu C, Calway T, Yuan C-S, et al. Epigallocatechin Gallate (EGCG) is the most effective cancer chemopreventive polyphenol in green tea. Nutrients. 2012;**4**(11):1679-1691

[25] Na H-K, Surh Y-J. Modulation of Nrf2-mediated antioxidant and detoxifying enzyme induction by the green tea polyphenol EGCG. Food and Chemical Toxicology. 2008;**46**(4):1271-1278

[26] Bushman JL. Green tea and cancer in humans: A review of the literature. Nutrition and Cancer. 1998;**31**(3):151-159

[27] Nakachi K, Matsuyama S, Miyake S, Suganuma M, Imai K. Preventive effects of drinking green tea on cancer and cardiovascular disease: Epidemiological evidence for multiple targeting prevention. BioFactors. 2000;**13**(1-4):49-54

[28] Suganuma M, Okabe S, Sueoka N, Sueoka E, Matsuyama S, Imai K, et al. Green tea and cancer chemoprevention. Mutation Research/Fundamental and Molecular Mechanisms of Mutagenesis. 1999;**428**(1-2):339-344

[29] Bocci V, Valacchi G. Free radicals and antioxidants: How to reestablish redox homeostasis in chronic diseases? Current Medicinal Chemistry. 2013;**20**(27):3397-3415

[30] Kuriyama S, Shimazu T, Ohmori K, Kikuchi N, Nakaya N, Nishino Y, et al. Green tea consumption and mortality due to cardiovascular disease, cancer, and all causes in Japan: The Ohsaki study. JAMA. 2006;**296**(10):1255-1265

[31] Sheikhzadeh N, Nofouzi K, Delazar A, Oushani AK. Immunomodulatory effects of decaffeinated green tea (Camellia sinensis) on the immune system of rainbow trout (Oncorhynchus mykiss). Fish & Shellfish Immunology. 2011;**31**(6):1268-1269

[32] Yang CS, Wang X. Green tea and cancer prevention. Nutrition and Cancer. 2010;**62**(7):931-937

[33] Basu A, Lucas EA. Mechanisms and effects of green tea on cardiovascular health. Nutrition Reviews. 2007;**65**(8):361-375

[34] Velayutham P, Babu A, Liu D. Green tea catechins and cardiovascular health:

An update. Current Medicinal Chemistry. 2008;**15**(18):1840

[35] Mann JI. Diet and risk of coronary heart disease and type 2 diabetes. The Lancet. 2002;**360**(9335):783-789

[36] Yusuf S, Reddy S, Ôunpuu S, Anand S. Global burden of cardiovascular diseases: Part II: Variations in cardiovascular disease by specific ethnic groups and geographic regions and prevention strategies. Circulation. 2001;**104**(23):2855-2864

[37] Kokubo Y, Iso H, Saito I, Yamagishi K, Yatsuya H, Ishihara J, et al. The impact of green tea and coffee consumption on the reduced risk of stroke incidence in Japanese population: The Japan public health center-based study cohort. Stroke. 2013;**44**(5):1369-1374

[38] Hodgson JM, Puddey IB, Burke V, Beilin LJ, Jordan N. Effects on blood pressure of drinking green and black tea. Journal of Hypertension. 1999;**17**(4):457-463

[39] Azam S, Hadi N, Khan NU, Hadi SM. Prooxidant property of green tea polyphenols epicatechin and epigallocatechin-3-gallate: Implications for anticancer properties. Toxicology In Vitro. 2004;**18**(5):555-561

[40] Cooper R, Morré DJ, Morré DM. Medicinal benefits of green tea: Part II. Review of anticancer properties. Journal of Alternative & Complementary Medicine. 2005;**11**(4):639-652

[41] Peng G, Dixon DA, Muga SJ, Smith TJ, Wargovich MJ. Green tea polyphenol (−)-epigallocatechin-3-gallate inhibits cyclooxygenase-2 expression in colon carcinogenesis. Molecular Carcinogenesis: Published in cooperation with the University of Texas MD Anderson Cancer Center. 2006;**45**(5):309-319

[42] Yoshizawa S, Horiuchi T, Fujiki H, Yoshida T, Okuda T, Sugimura T. Antitumor promoting activity of (−)-epigallocatechin gallate, the main constituent of "tannin" in green tea. Phytotherapy Research. 1987;**1**(1):44-47

[43] Andreasson A, Hagström H, Sköldberg F, Önnerhag K, Carlsson AC, Schmidt PT, et al. The prediction of colorectal cancer using anthropometric measures: A Swedish population-based cohort study with 22 years of follow-up. United European Gastroenterology Journal. 2019;7(9):1250-1260

[44] Shimizu M, Fukutomi Y, Ninomiya M, Nagura K, Kato T, Araki H, et al. Green tea extracts for the prevention of metachronous colorectal adenomas: A pilot study. Cancer Epidemiology and Prevention Biomarkers. 2008;**17**(11):3020-3025

[45] Makiuchi T, Sobue T, Kitamura T, Ishihara J, Sawada N, Iwasaki M, et al. Association between green tea/coffee consumption and biliary tract cancer: A population-based cohort study in Japan. Cancer Science. 2016;**107**(1):76-83

[46] Senggunprai L, Kukongviriyapan V, Prawan A, Kukongviriyapan U. Quercetin and EGCG exhibit chemopreventive effects in cholangiocarcinoma cells via suppression of JAK/STAT signaling pathway. Phytotherapy Research. 2014;**28**(6):841-848

[47] Fujiki H, Sueoka E, Watanabe T, Suganuma M. Synergistic enhancement of anticancer effects on numerous human cancer cell lines treated with the combination of EGCG, other green tea catechins, and anticancer compounds. Journal of Cancer Research and Clinical Oncology. 2015;**141**(9):1511-1522

[48] Panda D, Sharma A, Shukla NK, Jaiswal R, Dwivedi S, Raina V, et al. Gall bladder cancer and the role of dietary and lifestyle factors. European Journal of Cancer Prevention. 2013;**22**(5):431-437

[49] Panda D, Sharma A, Shukla NK, Jaiswal R, Dwivedi S, Raina V, et al. Gall bladder cancer and the role of dietary and lifestyle factors: A case-control study in a north Indian population. European Journal of Cancer Prevention. 2013;**22**(5):431-437. DOI: 10.1097/CEJ.0b013e32835f3b45

[50] Khaerunnisa S, Kurniawan H, Awaluddin R, Suhartati S, Soetjipto S. Potential inhibitor of COVID-19 main protease (Mpro) from several medicinal plant compounds by molecular docking study. Preprint. 2020;**2020**:2020030226

[51] Yang F, Zhang Y, Tariq A, Jiang X, Ahmed Z, Zhihao Z, et al. Food as medicine: A possible preventive measure against coronavirus disease (COVID-19). Phytotherapy Research. 2020;**34**(12):3124-3136

[52] Weng C-J, Yen G-C. Chemopreventive effects of dietary phytochemicals against cancer invasion and metastasis: Phenolic acids, monophenol, polyphenol, and their derivatives. Cancer Treatment Reviews. 2012;**38**(1):76-87

[53] Yang CS, Wang X, Lu G, Picinich SC. Cancer prevention by tea: Animal studies, molecular mechanisms and human relevance. Nature Reviews Cancer. 2009;**9**(6):429-439

[54] Ohgitani E, Shin-Ya M, Ichitani M, Kobayashi M, Takihara T, Kawamoto M, et al. Significant inactivation of SARS-CoV-2 in vitro by a green tea catechin, a catechin-derivative, and black tea galloylated theaflavins. Molecules. 2021;**26**(12):3572. DOI: 10.3390/molecules26123572

[55] Gokulakrisnan A, Jayachandran Dare B, Thirunavukkarasu C. Attenuation of the cardiac inflammatory changes and lipid anomalies by (−)-epigallocatechin-gallate in cigarette smoke-exposed rats. Molecular and Cellular Biochemistry. 2011;**354**(1):1-10

[56] Kim SJ, Li M, Jeong CW, Bae HB, Kwak SH, Lee SH, et al. Epigallocatechin-3-gallate, a green tea catechin, protects the heart against regional ischemia–reperfusion injuries through activation of risk survival pathways in rats. Archives of Pharmacal Research. 2014;**37**(8):1079-1085

[57] Jakubczyk K, Kochman J, Kwiatkowska A, Kałduńska J, Dec K, Kawczuga D, et al. Antioxidant properties and nutritional composition of matcha green tea. Food. 2020;**9**(4):483

[58] Bae J, Kim N, Shin Y, Kim S-Y, Kim Y-J. Activity of catechins and their applications. Biomedical Dermatology. 2020;**4**(1):1-10

[59] Ghosh R, Chakraborty A, Biswas A, Chowdhuri S. Evaluation of green tea polyphenols as novel corona virus (SARS CoV-2) main protease (Mpro) inhibitors–an in silico docking and molecular dynamics simulation study. Journal of Biomolecular Structure and Dynamics. 2021;**39**(12):4362-4374

[60] Lin Y-T, Wu Y-H, Tseng C-K, Lin C-K, Chen W-C, Hsu Y-C, et al. Green tea phenolic epicatechins inhibit hepatitis C virus replication via cycloxygenase-2 and attenuate virus-induced inflammation. PLoS One. 2013;**8**(1):e54466

[61] Mahmood MS, Mártinez JL, Aslam A, Rafique A, Vinet R, Laurido C, et al. Antiviral effects of green tea (Camellia sinensis) against pathogenic viruses in human and animals (a mini-review). African Journal of Traditional,

Complementary and Alternative Medicines. 2016;**13**(2):176-184

[62] Jang M, Park YI, Cha YE, Park R, Namkoong S, Lee JI, et al. Tea polyphenols EGCG and theaflavin inhibit the activity of SARS-CoV-2 3CL-protease in vitro. Evidence-Based Complementary and Alternative Medicine. 16 Sep 2020;**2020**:5630838. DOI: 10.1155/2020/5630838. PMID: 32963564; PMCID: PMC7499281

[63] Levy E, Delvin E, Marcil V, Spahis S. Can phytotherapy with polyphenols serve as a powerful approach for the prevention and therapy tool of novel coronavirus disease 2019 (COVID-19)? American Journal of Physiology-Endocrinology and Metabolism. 2020;**319**(4):E689-E708

[64] Menegazzi M, Campagnari R, Bertoldi M, Crupi R, Di Paola R, Cuzzocrea S. Protective effect of epigallocatechin-3-gallate (EGCG) in diseases with uncontrolled immune activation: Could such a scenario be helpful to counteract COVID-19? International Journal of Molecular Sciences. 2020;**21**(14):5171

[65] Mhatre S, Srivastava T, Naik S, Patravale V. Antiviral activity of green tea and black tea polyphenols in prophylaxis and treatment of COVID-19: A review. Phytomedicine. 2021;**85**:153286

[66] Sodagari HR, Bahramsoltani R, Farzaei MH, Abdolghaffari AH, Rezaei N, Taylor-Robinson AW. Tea polyphenols as natural products for potential future management of HIV infection-an overview. Journal of Natural Remedies. 2016;**16**(2):60-72

[67] Zhu Y, Xie DY. Docking characterization and in vitro inhibitory activity of flavan-3-ols and dimeric proanthocyanidins against the main protease activity of SARS-Cov-2. Frontiers in Plant Science. 30 Nov 2020;**11**:601316. DOI: 10.3389/fpls.2020.601316. PMID: 33329667; PMCID: PMC7733993

[68] Nguyen TTH, Woo H-J, Kang H-K, Nguyen VD, Kim Y-M, Kim D-W, et al. Flavonoid-mediated inhibition of SARS coronavirus 3C-like protease expressed in Pichia pastoris. Biotechnology Letters. 2012;**34**(5):831-838

[69] Ohishi T, Goto S, Monira P, Isemura M, Nakamura Y. Anti-inflammatory action of green tea. Anti-Inflammatory & Anti-Allergy Agents in Medicinal Chemistry (Formerly Current Medicinal Chemistry-Anti-Inflammatory and Anti-Allergy Agents). 2016;**15**(2):74-90

[70] Shan D, Fang Y, Ye Y, Liu J. EGCG reducing the susceptibility to cholesterol gallstone formation through the regulation of inflammation. Biomedicine & Pharmacotherapy. 2008;**62**(10):677-683

[71] Alzoubi KH, Mhaidat NM, Obaid EA, Khabour OF. Caffeine prevents memory impairment induced by hyperhomocysteinemia. Journal of Molecular Neuroscience. 2018;**66**(2):222-228

[72] Arendash GW, Mori T, Cao C, Mamcarz M, Runfeldt M, Dickson A, et al. Caffeine reverses cognitive impairment and decreases brain amyloid-β levels in aged Alzheimer's disease mice. Journal of Alzheimer's Disease. 2009;**17**(3):661-680

[73] Ritchie K, Carrière I, De Mendonca A, Portet F, Dartigues J-F, Rouaud O, et al. The neuroprotective effects of caffeine: A prospective population study (the three City study). Neurology. 2007;**69**(6):536-545

[74] Ullah F, Ali T, Ullah N, Kim MO. Caffeine prevents d-galactose-induced cognitive deficits, oxidative stress, neuroinflammation and neurodegeneration in the adult rat brain. Neurochemistry International. 2015;**90**:114-124

[75] Ettcheto M, Cano A, Manzine PR, Busquets O, Verdaguer E, Castro-Torres RD, et al. Epigallocatechin-3-Gallate (EGCG) improves cognitive deficits aggravated by an obesogenic diet through modulation of unfolded protein response in APPswe/PS1dE9 mice. Molecular Neurobiology. 2020;**57**(4):1814-1827

[76] Kim J, Funayama S, Izuo N, Shimizu T. Dietary supplementation of a high-temperature-processed green tea extract attenuates cognitive impairment in PS2 and Tg2576 mice. Bioscience, Biotechnology, and Biochemistry. 2019;**83**(12):2364-2371

[77] Kochman J, Jakubczyk K, Antoniewicz J, Mruk H, Janda K. Health benefits and chemical composition of matcha green tea: A review. Molecules. 2020;**26**(1):85

[78] Chu C, Deng J, Man Y, Qu Y. Green tea extracts Epigallocatechin-3-gallate for different treatments. BioMed Research International. 2017;**2017**:5615647. DOI: 10.1155/2017/5615647

[79] Kasper B, Salameh A, Krausch M, Kiefer P, Kostelka M, Mohr FW, et al. Epigallocatechin gallate attenuates cardiopulmonary bypass–associated lung injury. Journal of Surgical Research. 2016;**201**(2):313-325

[80] Salameh A, Dhein S, Mewes M, Sigusch S, Kiefer P, Vollroth M, et al. Anti-oxidative or anti-inflammatory additives reduce ischemia/reperfusions injury in an animal model of cardiopulmonary bypass. Saudi Journal of Biological Sciences. 2020;**27**(1):18-29

[81] Mahajan N, Dhawan V, Sharma G, Jain S, Kaul D. Induction of inflammatory gene expression by THP-1 macrophages cultured in normocholesterolaemic hypertensive sera and modulatory effects of green tea polyphenols. Journal of Human Hypertension. 2008;**22**(2):141-143

[82] Kolahdouzan M, Hamadeh MJ. The neuroprotective effects of caffeine in neurodegenerative diseases. CNS Neuroscience & Therapeutics. 2017;**23**(4):272-290

Chapter 2

Green Tea as An Ingredient in Food Combinations Provide Metabolic Improvements

Alexandra Becraft and Neil Shay

Abstract

The objective of the studies summarized in the present chapter was to determine if intake of walnuts alone or in combination with two or more other phytochemical-rich foods would ameliorate some of the negative metabolic effects developed from consumption of an obesogenic and diabetogenic, Western-style diet. The two studies summarized in this chapter were designed the same using a C57BL/6 J mouse strain as a model to induce obesity using a high fat, sugar, and cholesterol diet, while supplementing the diet with 1.5 servings/day of various nutrient-dense whole foods. In Part 1, walnut alone and walnut plus green tea supplementation were studied. Based on the results of Part 1, Part 2 studied supplementation with four whole foods (walnut, green tea, cherry, and red raspberry) in combination to determine any synergistic effects. In both studies, the combination of two or more test foods appeared to work synergistically to produce further changes in metabolism than compared to walnuts alone. Key findings included attenuation of weight gain, improved circulating serum insulin and cytokine concentrations, improved hepatic levels of protective omega-3 polyunsaturated fatty acids, as well as decreased levels of hepatic proinflammatory fatty acids.

Keywords: obesity, high-fat diet, phytochemicals, walnut, green tea, cherry, raspberry

1. Introduction

Consumption of phytochemical-rich foods has been shown to ameliorate some of the negative metabolic effects resulting from consumption of an obesogenic and diabetogenic, Western-style diet. Specifically, green tea contains a series of polyphenols known as catechins, mainly epigallocatechin gallate (EGCG), epicatechin gallate, and gallocatechin gallate [1]. Many of the demonstrated beneficial effects of green tea are attributed to its most abundant catechin, EGCG. One study demonstrated that EGCG treatment suppressed hyperglycemia, proteinuria, and lipid peroxidation. These results also suggested that EGCG may alleviate renal damage caused by abnormal glucose metabolism-associated oxidative stress [2]. Epigallocatechin gallate may also modulate appetite and reduce food intake [3, 4]. Furthermore, green tea catechin consumption has been shown to stimulate hepatic lipid metabolism, through mechanisms such as increased acyl-CoA oxidase and β-oxidation activity [1], as well as stimulate O_2 consumption and energy expenditure [5].

These recent studies demonstrating the therapeutic potential of consuming green tea catechins have led to an interest in consuming green tea and green tea extract to remediate metabolic dysfunction. Green tea extract has been reported to stimulate brown adipose tissue thermogenesis along with fat oxidation. It was suggested that green tea's thermogenic effect may be stimulated through the interaction of its high catechin and caffeine content with sympathetically released noradrenaline [6]. In addition, a meta-analysis conducted in 2015, demonstrated that green tea drinkers have a reduced risk of liver disease including liver steatosis [7]. Epidemiological studies have also suggested that regular consumption of five to six or more cups of green tea per day has pronounced cardiovascular and metabolic health benefits [8].

It is thought that some phytochemical-rich foods may work synergistically to remediate metabolic syndrome when consumed together. Such foods of interest are fruits like red raspberries and cherries along with polyunsaturated fatty acid-rich nuts like walnuts. Cherries are rich in anthocyanins and have been previously observed to improve glucose tolerance and liver lipid accumulation [9], while bioactive polyphenols present in red raspberries may remediate oxidative stress and inflammation [10]. Walnuts have been shown to improve serum lipid levels as well as other cardiovascular parameters [11].

Part 1 of this chapter summarizes research demonstrating the changes to metabolism when consuming an obesigenic high-fat diet supplemented with walnut alone and walnut plus green tea. Some results from Part 1 were previously published, see [12]. Part 2 adds to the results from Part 1 by including a second study where four whole foods (whole cherry and red raspberry along with walnut and green tea) were consumed together to determine their synergistic effect, if any, on remediating metabolic syndrome, again, in the context of a high-fat diet provided to male mice. Both Part 1 and Part 2 studies were designed the same using a C57BL/6 J mouse strain as a model to induce obesity and study the negative metabolic effects that develop when presented with a high-calorie Western-style diet. The hypotheses of both studies were that consumption of the test foods would work to remediate metabolic complications in C57BL/6 J male mice fed a high-fat, high-sucrose, and high-cholesterol diet modeling an obesigenic and diabetogenic Western-style diet.

2. Part 1: effect of walnut and synergistic effect of walnut plus green tea consumption

A rodent model using C57BL/6 J mice fed an obesogenic and diabetogenic high fat diet with added sucrose and cholesterol was designed to evaluate changes in metabolism when supplemented with walnut (W) or walnut plus green tea (W + GT). Walnuts were provided in the diets as ground nuts and the green tea was a dried powder derived from an aqueous extract of dried green tea leaves (Triarco Industries). Diets were formulated to mimic a typical 2000 kcal/day diet with whole walnuts added at an equivalence to 1.5 servings per day and green tea added at 1% (wt:wt), which is consistent with normal human intake levels shown in other rodent studies [13].

The final body weight of the HF diet group provided with walnuts alone did not significantly differ from the HF-fed control. However, the group supplemented with

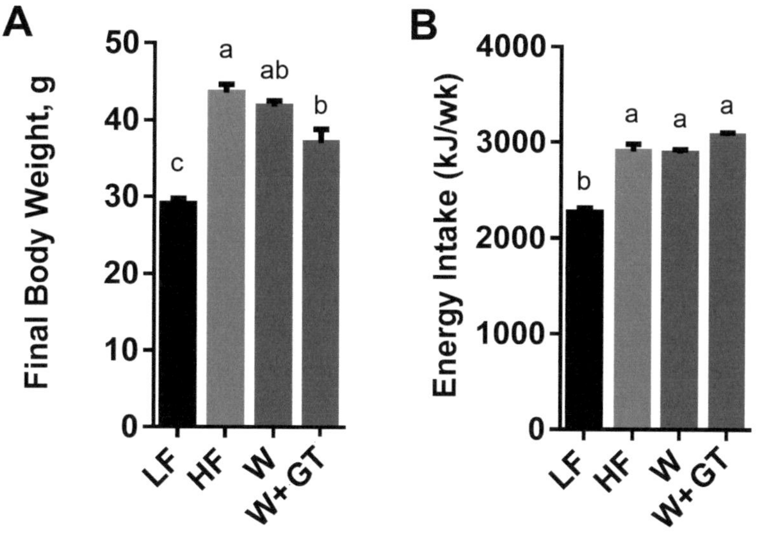

Figure 1.
Final body weight (A) and energy intake (B) of obese male mice fed a LF or HF diet alone or one that included walnuts alone or walnut plus green tea for 9 weeks. Values are means ± SEMs, n = 8 mice. One-way ANOVA indicated significant differences between diet groups (p ≤ 0.05). Values that do not share a letter differ (p ≤ 0.05).

additional green tea (W + GT) was significantly lower than the HF-fed control group ($p \leq 0.05$), despite consuming a similar amount of energy (**Figure 1A** and **B**). This result is consistent with other findings demonstrating that green tea polyphenols, specifically (−)-epigallocatechin-3-gallate, may have protective effects against obesity by increasing thermogenesis [14–17].

Metabolomic analysis comparing 594 different hepatic biochemicals detected in liver samples from the mice in each of the diet groups showed several metabolomic changes, including changes in metabolites related to energetics, inflammation, and redox homeostasis. The W + GT supplemented group showed significant increases in S-methylmethionine, when compared to both HF ($p \leq 0.05$) and LF ($p \leq 0.05$) control groups and the W supplemented group ($p \leq 0.05$). S-methylmethionine is a plant-derived metabolite that can be used as a carbon source for bacterial growth [18] which may imply beneficial effects on the host microbiome with supplementation of green tea. Additionally, increases in xanthine metabolites (e.g., paraxanthine, theobromine, theophylline) in the W + GT supplemented group compared to both the HF ($p \leq 0.05$) and LF ($p \leq 0.05$) control groups and the W supplemented group ($p \leq 0.05$) were observed. This result likely reflects naturally occurring xanthine metabolites in GT as well as liver metabolism of increased caffeine intake from GT extract using the cytochrome P450 system.

The omega-3 polyunsaturated fatty acid linolenate was also elevated in the walnut-supplemented diets, which may indicate potential relevance to inflammation. Both the W and W + GT groups showed significant increases in omega-3 polyunsaturated fatty acids, eicosapentaenoate (EPA), and docosapentaenoate (DPA), compared to LF and HF control groups (**Figure 2**) These results suggest that walnut and green tea supplementation may negatively regulate inflammation. However, increases in docosapentaenoate (DHA) were not significantly altered. These results are consistent with previous studies reporting that increased ALA consumption (herein via walnut)

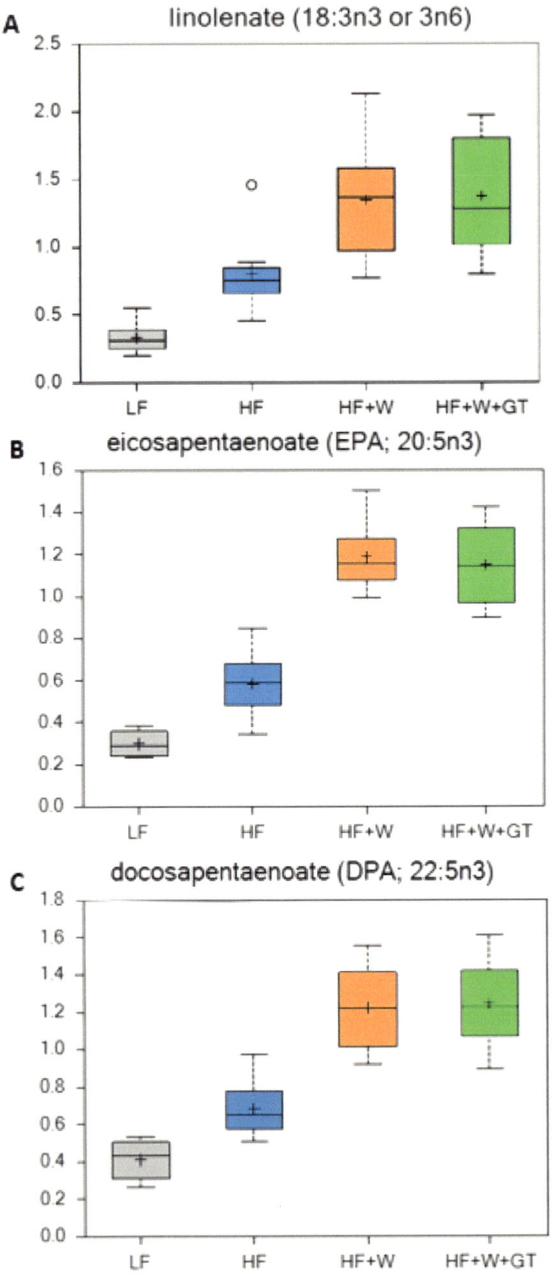

Figure 2.
Box plots demonstrating metabolomic analysis of livers of obese male mice fed a LF or HF diet alone or one that included walnuts alone or walnut plus green tea for 9 weeks.

results in little to no change in DHA plasma lipid fractions, as large amounts of ALA are required to endogenously convert to significant levels of DHA [19–24].

Supplementation with walnuts alone did not result in significant changes to detected eicosanoids when compared to HF control but did show non-significant trends toward decreased prostaglandin F2alpha ($p \leq 0.10$) and 12-hydroxyeicosatetraenoic acid (HETE) such that it was statistically indistinguishable from the LF

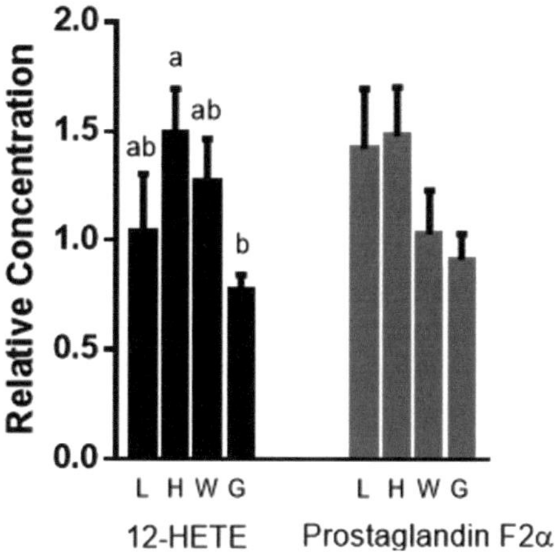

Figure 3.
Relative concentration of hepatic proinflammatory fatty acids in obese male mice fed a LF or HF diet alone or one that included walnuts alone or walnut plus green tea for 9 weeks. Values are means ± SEMs, n = 8 mice. One-way ANOVA indicated significant differences between diet groups (p ≤ 0.05). Values that do not share a letter differ (p ≤ 0.05). G, walnuts plus green tea; H, high fat, HETE, hydroxyeicosatetraenoic acid; L, low fat; W, walnuts.

control group (**Figure 3**). However, W + GT, compared to HF control, showed a significant decrease in 12-HETE, suggestive of declining inflammation. These results are consistent with serum cytokine concentrations measured of MCP-1, giving additional insight into the secretion and recruitment of activated immune cells in supplemented mice. MCP-1 concentrations were elevated with consumption of a HF diet compared to LF diet ($p \leq 0.05$); however, the addition of walnut reduced MCP-1 such that it was intermediate to the LF and HF control groups and statistically indistinguishable from the levels measured in the LF group (data not shown). The addition of green tea to the walnut diet resulted in even further lowering of MCP-1 levels, such that they were statistically equivalent to the LF control group (data not shown). Of note, measured concentrations of TNFα and IL-6 were both measured and saw no significant decreases in HF + W group, but significant elevation of IL-6 was observed in W + GT group ($p \leq 0.05$) (data not shown).

3. Part 2: synergistic effects of cherry, red raspberry, walnut, and green tea (CRWG)

The synergistic effects of consuming whole cherry, raspberry, walnut, and green tea in combination were determined in an independent study. The same rodent model as Part 1, C57Bl/6 J mice consuming an obesogenic and diabetogenic high fat diet with added sucrose and cholesterol, was used to evaluate the synergistic impact of these four foods on metabolism and microbiome of the ceca.

Despite consuming similar amounts of energy, the mice supplemented with HF + CRWG had lower final body weight and change in body weight compared to the HF diet alone (**Figure 4A** and **B**). This result is consistent with previous studies on cherry, raspberry, and walnut consumption and reduced weight gain [25–30]. Additionally, walnut and green tea consumption have been demonstrated to increase resting energy expenditure and thermogenesis, which may be a potential mechanism through which decreased weight gain occurred [6, 31]. Elevation of food efficiency in

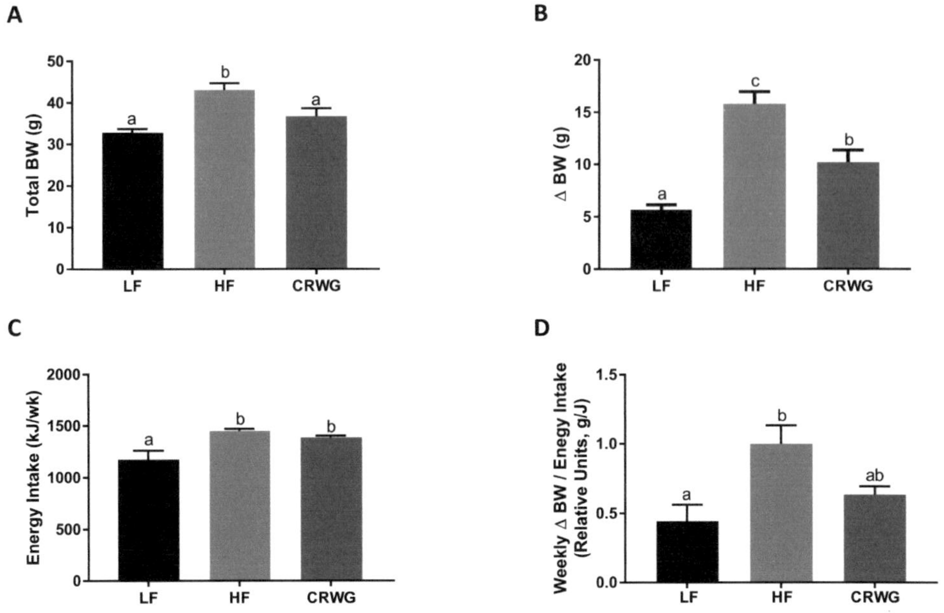

Figure 4.
Total body weight (A) net change in body weight, (B) average weekly energy intake, (C) energy efficiency, (D) of male C57BL/6 J mice fed either a low fat (LF) diet, a high fat (HF) diet alone, or HF plus cherry, raspberry, walnut, and green tea (CRWG) after 10 weeks. One-way ANOVA indicated significant differences between diet groups ($p \leq 0.05$). Values that do not share a letter differ ($p \leq 0.05$).

HF-fed mice was also attenuated with the addition of CRWG to the diet (**Figure 4D**). This observation suggests that, although the CRWG group ate similar amounts of energy as the HF control, the CRWG group was less efficient in converting the diet to energy compared to the HF-fed control. Again, this result may be due to increased thermogenesis initiated by the green tea and walnut consumption.

Fasting blood glucose was measured in weeks 9 and 10. Treatment groups fed HF supplemented with CRWG had a slightly reduced fasting blood glucose, but it was not statistically significant from the HF-fed control group (**Figure 5A**). In addition, results from an insulin sensitivity test performed in week 10 showed the HF + CRWG treatment group was not statistically different from the HF-fed control group (data not shown). However, serum collected from the mice at necropsy was used to perform an ELISA to quantify circulating serum insulin, which was indeed reduced with HF + CRWG supplementation compared to HF diet alone such that it was statistically indistinguishable from the LF control mice (**Figure 5B**). Insulin secretion by β-cells increases in response to insulin resistance to moderate elevated blood glucose [32]. Therefore, initial upregulation of β-cell function in response to a HF diet may be regulated with CRWG supplementation as evidenced by reduced serum insulin concentrations compared to HF diet alone. The HOMA-IR and HOMA-%β calculations support this conclusion, as the HF-fed control mice were assessed to have greater development of insulin resistance and heightened β-cell function compared to the HF + CRWG treatment group (**Figure 5C** and **D**). Tart cherry extracts have been shown to increase nitric oxide (NO) production in cell and animal models [33, 34]. Similarly, (−)-epicatechin, found in green tea, may help maintain healthy blood pressure ranges when consumed with HF diet via restoration of NO bioavailability [35]. Increased NO production may improve insulin sensitivity and decrease glucose

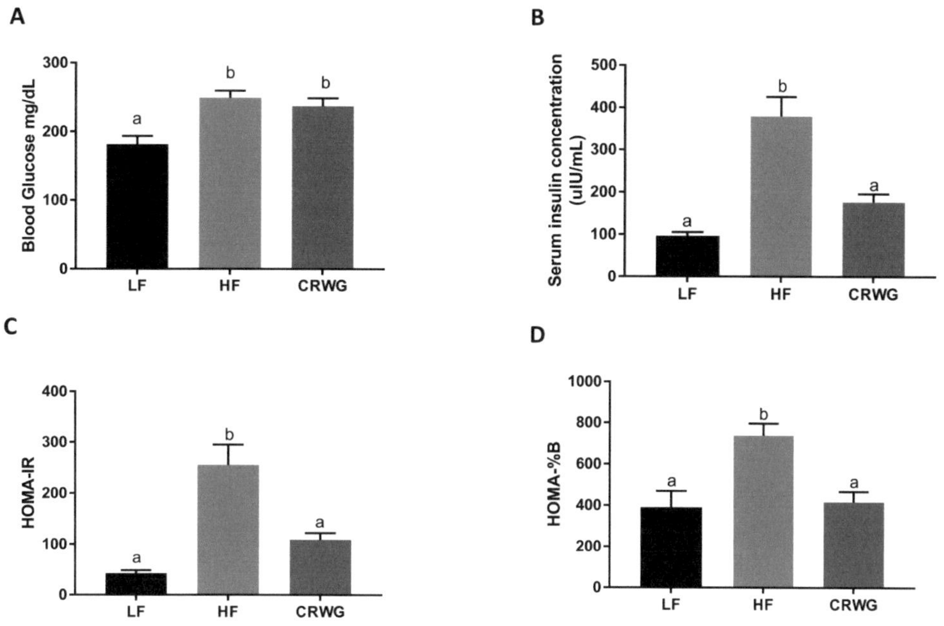

Figure 5.
Average fasting blood glucose concentration at week 9 and week 10 (A) serum insulin concentration, (B) homeostasis model assessment of insulin resistance (HOMA-IR), (C) and homeostatic model assessment of β-cell function (HOMA-%β), (D) of male C57BL/6 J mice fed either a low fat (LF) diet, a high fat (HF) diet alone, or HF plus cherry, raspberry, walnut, and green tea (CRWG) after 10 weeks. One-way ANOVA indicated significant differences between diet groups ($p \leq 0.05$). Values that do not share a letter differ ($p \leq 0.05$).

Tissue weights	Diet groups[2]		
	LF	HF	HF + CRWG
Liver (g)	1.1 ± 0.08[a]	2.24 ± 0.25[b]	1.55 ± 0.16[ab]
Liver/body weight (g/g, %)	3.37 ± 0.17[a]	4.89 ± 0.35[b]	4.17 ± 0.23[ab]

[1]*Values are expressed as means ± SEM of each group, values that do not share a letter differ ($p \leq 0.05$).*
[2]*Low fat diet (LF), high fat diet (HF), or HF plus cherry, raspberry, walnut, and green tea (HF + CRWG).*

Table 1.
Organ tissue weights and weights as percentage of final body weight of male C57BL/6 J mice[1].

concentrations via NO-mediated increases in blood flow, resulting in more efficient uptake of glucose by skeletal muscle [36–38]. Therefore, insulin sensitivity and β-cell function may have been improved by CRWG supplementation because of increased NO production from the tart cherry and green tea components of the diet.

Liver weight to body weight ratios were measured postmortem (**Table 1**). Liver weight and liver weight to body weight ratio of HF-fed control group was significantly higher than the LF-fed mice, while liver weight and liver weight to body weight ratio of HF + CRWG treatment group was reduced such that it was statistically indistinguishable from the LF-fed control group. Additionally, stained cross sections of the liver tissue were used to identify liver lipid accumulation in each group. A representative image for each group is shown in **Figure 6**. White globules are indicative of lipid accumulation, red staining indicates cytosol, and

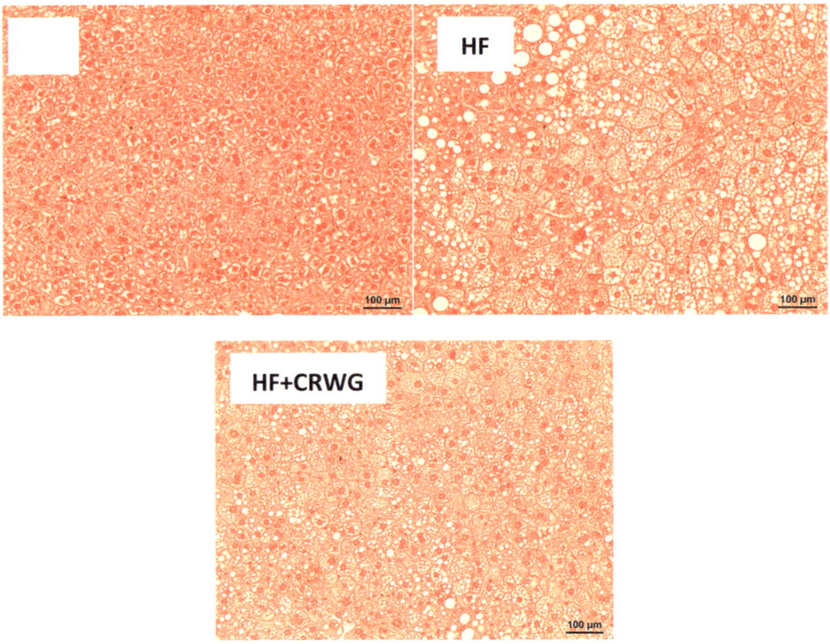

Figure 6.
Hematoxylin–eosin stained liver cross sections of male C57BL/6 J mice fed either a low fat (LF) diet, a high fat (HF) diet alone, or HF plus cherry, raspberry, walnut, and green tea (CRWG) after 10 weeks. Slides were observed under 400x magnification (40x objective) using Nikon Eclipse 50i microscope (Nikon Corporation, Tokyo, Japan) equipped with an Infinity 1-3C camera (Lumenera Corporation, Ottawa, ON, Canada).

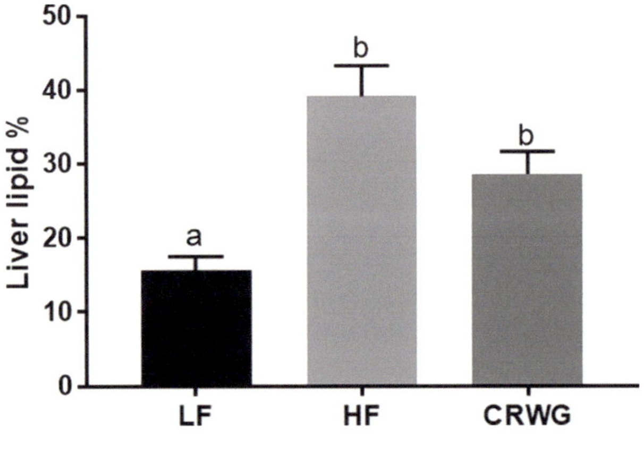

Figure 7.
Liver lipid percentage of hematoxylin–eosin-stained liver cross sections of male C57BL/6 J mice fed either a low fat (LF) diet, a high fat (HF) diet alone, or HF plus cherry, raspberry, walnut, and green tea (CRWG) after 10 weeks. One-way ANOVA indicated significant differences between diet groups ($p \leq 0.05$). Values that do not share a letter differ ($p \leq 0.05$).

dark red circles are the nuclei. Analysis of lipid percentage within the hepatocytes of each group is shown in **Figure** 7. Although not significant, HF + CRWG diet did appear to reduce liver lipid accumulation by approximately 30% compared to HF diet alone. Typically, liver weight increases proportionally to body weight gain, thus these results may suggest potential improvement in liver lipid accumulation in the CRWG supplemented mice.

Bacteria type[2] (%)	Diet groups[3]		
	LF	HF	HF + CRWG
k_Bacteria p_Bacteroidetes c_Bacteroidia o_Bacteroidales f_S24–7	38.2 ± 3.2[b]	21.0 ± 1.2[a]	25.3 ± 3.2[a]
k_Bacteria p_Verrucomicrobia c_Verrucomicrobiae o_Verrucomicrobiales f_*Verrucomicrobiaceae* g_*Akkermansia* s_*muciniphila*	11.9 ± 1.6[a]	26.1 ± 2.5[b]	17.7 ± 2.8[a]
k_Bacteria p_Firmicutes c_Clostridia o_Clostridiales	14.1 ± 2.0	14.7 ± 0.8	14.9 ± 1.0
k_Bacteria p_Firmicutes c_Clostridia o_Clostridiales f_*Ruminococcaceae*‡	7.3 ± 1.3[ab]	11.4 ± 1.4[b]	5.9 ± 0.8[a]
k_Bacteria p_Bacteroidetes c_Bacteroidia o_Bacteroidales f_*Bacteroidaceae* g_*Bacteroides*	4.8 ± 0.6[a]	6.3 ± 0.6[a]	19.7 ± 2.3[b]
k_Bacteria p_Firmicutes c_Clostridia o_Clostridiales f_*Ruminococcaceae*‡	4.3 ± 0.5[a]	7.7 ± 0.7[b]	3.8 ± 0.5[a]
k_Bacteria p_Firmicutes c_Clostridia o_Clostridiales f_*Lachnospiraceae*	5.9 ± 1.2[b]	2.0 ± 0.2[a]	3.3 ± 0.4[ab]

[1]*Values are expressed as means ± SEM of each group, values that do not share a letter differ ($p \leq 0.05$).*
[2]*Some populations sequenced were not complete down to the lowest taxonomic level due to incomplete sequences for these bacteria within the Greengenes database in QIIME2, and thus cannot be differentiated.*
[3]*Low fat diet (LF), high fat diet (HF), or HF plus cherry, raspberry, walnut, and green tea (HF + CRWG).*

Table 2.
Relative frequency of the top seven bacteria in the ceca[1].

The microbiome was quantified from the cecum of each mouse, and variation in the top seven most prolific gut bacteria of each group can be seen in **Table 2**. Among these bacteria, one group was from the phylum Bacteroidetes and family S24–7. This group of bacteria has previously been demonstrated to triple in number in HF diet fed mice that developed diabetes versus HF diet fed mice that were resistant to diabetes development [39]. Our findings showed that LF-fed animals had significantly higher number of S24–7 bacteria than any of the HF-fed groups, suggesting that these bacteria may be beneficial for maintaining a healthy metabolism. Another study found increased abundance of S24–7 bacteria following remission of colitis, again inferring a positive relationship within the host [40]. This variability between studies may be due to differences in diet formulation, animal model, and microbiome composition analysis and demonstrates the difficulty in reaching a scientific consensus on the beneficial and harmful effects of certain intestinal bacterial on metabolism. The second group of bacteria were from the genus Bacteroides, which have been reported to act commensally in the gut [41]. We observed a marked increase in Bacteroides in the HF + CRWG group such that it was significantly higher than both the LF and HF controls. Added fiber, especially from the raspberry component of the diet, may be a contributing factor to the increased frequency.

One of the bacteria analyzed was from the phylum Verrucomicrobia, specifically Akkermansia muciniphila (A. muciniphila). In the current study, we observed the highest degree of A. muciniphila proliferation in the HF control group, which is inconsistent with previous publications demonstrating its beneficial effect on weight maintenance and metabolism [42, 43]. Furthermore, other reports have showed that polyphenol intake promotes A. muciniphila growth; [44, 45] whereas, in the present study, CRWG fed mice had lower relative abundance than the HF-fed controls. The variability of our result with other literature could have been due to differences in diet administration and/or microbiome analysis.

Four of the analyzed bacteria belonged to the order Clostridiales from the phylum, Firmicutes. Members of this order have been previously associated with obesity; however, there is still vast variability within the lower taxonomic levels [43, 46, 47]. In our findings, we observed an increased shift in the frequency of two of the four Clostridiales bacteria in HF-fed mice. These two bacterial populations belonged to the family Ruminococcaceae. Supplementation with HF + CRWG resulted in reduced frequency of both Ruminococcaceae populations identified when compared to the HF diet alone. Alternatively, we observed a decrease in Clostridiales bacteria belonging to the family Lachnospiraceae in HF-fed mice. Supplementation with HF + CRWG resulted in increased frequency of this population. Increased proliferation of Lachnospiraceae with LF diet as well as polyphenol intake has been previously demonstrated [48]. Thus, our findings may suggest a positive intestinal shift in bacterial strains associated with both lean and obese phenotypes of Clostridiales bacteria with supplementation of CRWG.

4. Conclusions

Part 1: These data suggest that supplementation with walnut and walnut plus green tea provided at typical dietary levels may influence metabolism when consumed with a high-fat obesogenic Western-style diet. Specifically, supplementation with walnuts plus green tea may act synergistically to further decrease energy efficiency, improve levels of protective omega-3 polyunsaturated fatty acids, as well as decrease levels of hepatic proinflammatory fatty acids and cytokine markers of inflammation than walnuts alone.

Part 2: In obese male mice, modest level of dietary supplementation with cherry, raspberry, walnut, and green tea significantly improved circulating serum insulin concentrations and may protect against insulin resistance and heightened β-cell function. Our data suggests these foods may act synergistically to prevent the onset of metabolic syndrome. There was also profound attenuation of weight gain and food efficiency, suggesting that these four foods may act synergistically to help with weight maintenance. Future research investigating the synergistic effect of these four foods in a human trial would help further elucidate how these metabolic benefits translate to human consumption.

Acknowledgements

We thank the many laboratory colleagues who helped with animal husbandry and other technical tasks related to this project. Additionally, we are grateful to our colleague Jason Kinchen at University of Virginia for assistance in analysis of metabolomic data. Funding was provided in part by the California Walnut Commission. Green Tea powder was generously provided by Triarco Industries.

Conflict of interest

The authors declare no conflict of interest.

Author details

Alexandra Becraft* and Neil Shay*
Department of Food Science and Technology, Oregon State University, Corvallis, Oregon, USA

*Address all correspondence to: arbecraft@gmail.com and neil.shay@oregonstate.edu

References

[1] Murase T, Nagasawa A, Suzuki J, Hase T, Tokimitsu I. Beneficial effects of tea catechins on diet-induced obesity: Stimulation of lipid catabolism in the liver. International Journal of Obesity. Nov 2002;**26**(11):1459-1464

[2] Yamabe N, Yokozawa T, Oya T, Kim M. Therapeutic potential of (−)-epigallocatechin 3-O-gallate on renal damage in diabetic nephropathy model rats. The Journal of Pharmacology and Experimental Therapeutics. 1 Oct 2006;**319**(1):228-236

[3] Kao YH, Hiipakka RA, Liao S. Modulation of endocrine systems and food intake by green tea epigallocatechin gallate. Endocrinology. 1 Mar 2000;**141**(3):980-987

[4] Kao YH, Hiipakka RA, Liao S. Modulation of obesity by a green tea catechin. The American Journal of Clinical Nutrition. 1 Nov 2000;**72**(5):1232-1233

[5] Dulloo AG, Duret C, Rohrer D, Girardier L, Mensi N, Fathi M, et al. Efficacy of a green tea extract rich in catechin polyphenols and caffeine in increasing 24-h energy expenditure and fat oxidation in humans. The American Journal of Clinical Nutrition. 1 Dec 1999;**70**(6):1040-1045

[6] Dulloo AG, Seydoux J, Girardier L, Chantre P, Vandermander J. Green tea and thermogenesis: Interactions between catechin-polyphenols, caffeine and sympathetic activity. International Journal of Obesity. Feb 2000;**24**(2):252-258

[7] Yin X, Yang J, Li T, Song L, Han T, Yang M, et al. The effect of green tea intake on risk of liver disease: A meta analysis. International Journal of Clinical and Experimental Medicine. 2015;**8**(6):8339

[8] Wolfram S. Effects of green tea and EGCG on cardiovascular and metabolic health. Journal of the American College of Nutrition. 1 Aug 2007;**26**(4): 373S-388S

[9] Jayaprakasam B, Olson LK, Schutzki RE, Tai MH, Nair MG. Amelioration of obesity and glucose intolerance in high-fat-fed C57BL/6 mice by anthocyanins and ursolic acid in Cornelian cherry (*Cornus mas*). Journal of Agricultural and Food Chemistry. 11 Jan 2006;**54**(1):243-248

[10] Burton-Freeman BM, Sandhu AK, Edirisinghe I. Red raspberries and their bioactive polyphenols: Cardiometabolic and neuronal health links. Advances in Nutrition. Jan 2016;**7**(1):44-65

[11] Estruch R, Ros E, Salas-Salvadó J, Covas MI, Corella D, Arós F, et al. Primary prevention of cardiovascular disease with a Mediterranean diet. The New England Journal of Medicine. 4 Apr 2013;**368**(14):1279-1290

[12] Luo T, Miranda-Garcia O, Adamson A, Hamilton-Reeves J, Sullivan DK, Kinchen JM, et al. Consumption of walnuts in combination with other whole foods produces physiologic, metabolic, and gene expression changes in obese C57BL/6J high-fat–fed male mice. The Journal of Nutrition. 1 Sep 2016;**146**(9):1641-1650

[13] Bruno RS, Dugan CE, Smyth JA, DiNatale DA, Koo SI. Green tea extract protects leptin-deficient, spontaneously obese mice from hepatic steatosis and

injury. The Journal of Nutrition. 1 Feb 2008;**138**(2):323-331

[14] Lee MS, Shin Y, Jung S, Kim Y. Effects of epigallocatechin-3-gallate on thermogenesis and mitochondrial biogenesis in brown adipose tissues of diet-induced obese mice. Food & Nutrition Research. 1 Jan 2017;**61**(1):1325307

[15] Heber D, Zhang Y, Yang J, Ma JE, Henning SM, Li Z. Green tea, black tea, and oolong tea polyphenols reduce visceral fat and inflammation in mice fed high-fat, high-sucrose obesogenic diets. The Journal of Nutrition. 2014 Sep 1;**144**(9):1385-1393

[16] Sae-tan S, Rogers CJ, Lambert JD. Voluntary exercise and green tea enhance the expression of genes related to energy utilization and attenuate metabolic syndrome in high fat fed mice. Molecular Nutrition & Food Research. May 2014;**58**(5):1156-1159

[17] Ueda M, Ashida H. Green tea prevents obesity by increasing expression of insulin-like growth factor binding protein-1 in adipose tissue of high-fat diet-fed mice. Journal of Agricultural and Food Chemistry. 12 Sep 2012;**60**(36):8917-8923

[18] Thanbichler M, Neuhierl B, Böck A. S-methylmethionine metabolism in Escherichia coli. Journal of Bacteriology. 15 Jan 1999;**181**(2):662-665

[19] Hussein N, Ah-Sing E, Wilkinson P, Leach C, Griffin BA, Millward DJ. Long-chain conversion of [13C] linoleic acid and α-linolenic acid in response to marked changes in their dietary intake in men. Journal of Lipid Research. 1 Feb 2005;**46**(2):269-280

[20] Kelley DS, Nelson GJ, Love JE, Branch LB, Taylor PC, Schmidt PC, et al. Dietary alpha-linolenic acid alters tissue fatty acid composition, but not blood lipids, lipoproteins or coagulation status in humans. Lipids. 1993;**28**:533-537

[21] Mantzioris E, James MJ, Gibson RA, Cleland LG. Dietary substitution with an α-linolenic acid-rich vegetable oil increases eicosapentaenoic acid concentrations in tissues. The American Journal of Clinical Nutrition. 1 Jun 1994;**59**(6):1304-1309

[22] Valsta LM, Salminen I, Aro A, Mutanen M. Alpha-linolenic acid in rapeseed oil partly compensates for the effect of fish restriction on plasma long chain n-3 fatty acids. European Journal of Clinical Nutrition. 1 Apr 1996;**50**(4):229-235

[23] Finnegan YE, Minihane AM, Leigh-Firbank EC, Kew S, Meijer GW, Muggli R, et al. Plant-and marine-derived n-3 polyunsaturated fatty acids have differential effects on fasting and postprandial blood lipid concentrations and on the susceptibility of LDL to oxidative modification in moderately hyperlipidemic subjects. The American Journal of Clinical Nutrition. 1 Apr 2003;**77**(4):783-795

[24] Goyens PL, Spilker ME, Zock PL, Katan MB, Mensink RP. Conversion of α-linolenic acid in humans is influenced by the absolute amounts of α-linolenic acid and linoleic acid in the diet and not by their ratio. The American Journal of Clinical Nutrition. 1 Jun 2006;**84**(1):44-53

[25] Luo T, Miranda-Garcia O, Adamson A, Sasaki G, Shay NF. Development of obesity is reduced in high-fat fed mice fed whole raspberries, raspberry juice concentrate, and a combination of the raspberry phytochemicals ellagic acid and

raspberry ketone. Journal of Berry Research. 1 Jan 2016;**6**(2):213-223

[26] Luo T, Miranda-Garcia O, Sasaki G, Shay NF. Consumption of a single serving of red raspberries per day reduces metabolic syndrome parameters in high-fat fed mice. Food & Function. 2017;**8**(11):4081-4088

[27] Sabaté J, Cordero-MacIntyre Z, Siapco G, Torabian S, Haddad E. Does regular walnut consumption lead to weight gain? The British Journal of Nutrition. 2005 Nov;**94**(5):859-864

[28] Seymour EM, Lewis SK, Urcuyo-Llanes DE, Tanone II, Kirakosyan A, Kaufman PB, et al. Regular tart cherry intake alters abdominal adiposity, adipose gene transcription, and inflammation in obesity-prone rats fed a high fat diet. Journal of Medicinal Food. 1 Oct 2009;**12**(5):935-942

[29] Vadivel V, Kunyanga CN, Biesalski HK. Health benefits of nut consumption with special reference to body weight control. Nutrition. 1 Nov 2012;**28**(11-12):1089-1097

[30] Wu L, Piotrowski K, Rau T, Waldmann E, Broedl UC, Demmelmair H, et al. Walnut-enriched diet reduces fasting non-HDL-cholesterol and apolipoprotein B in healthy Caucasian subjects: A randomized controlled cross-over clinical trial. Metabolism. 1 Mar 2014;**63**(3):382-391

[31] Mattes RD, Dreher ML. Nuts and healthy body weight maintenance mechanisms. Asia Pacific Journal of Clinical Nutrition. Mar 2010;**19**(1):137-141

[32] Cerf ME. Beta cell dysfunction and insulin resistance. Frontiers in Endocrinology. Mar 2013;**27**(4):37

[33] Seeram NP, Momin RA, Nair MG, Bourquin LD. Cyclooxygenase inhibitory and antioxidant cyanidin glycosides in cherries and berries. Phytomedicine. 1 Jan 2001;**8**(5):362-369

[34] Wang H, Nair MG, Strasburg GM, Chang YC, Booren AM, Gray JI, et al. Antioxidant and antiinflammatory activities of anthocyanins and their aglycon, cyanidin, from tart cherries. Journal of Natural Products. 26 Feb 1999;**62**(2):294-296

[35] Litterio MC, Prieto MA, Adamo AM, Elesgaray R, Oteiza PI, Galleano M, et al. (−)-Epicatechin reduces blood pressure increase in high-fructose-fed rats: Effects on the determinants of nitric oxide bioavailability. The Journal of Nutritional Biochemistry. 1 Jul 2015;**26**(7):745-751

[36] Collins JK, Wu G, Perkins-Veazie P, Spears K, Claypool PL, Baker RA, et al. Watermelon consumption increases plasma arginine concentrations in adults. Nutrition. 1 Mar 2007;**23**(3):261-266

[37] Sansbury BE, Hill BG. Regulation of obesity and insulin resistance by nitric oxide. Free Radical Biology & Medicine. Aug 2014;**1**(73):383-399

[38] Wu G, Collins JK, Perkins-Veazie P, Siddiq M, Dolan KD, Kelly KA, et al. Dietary supplementation with watermelon pomace juice enhances arginine availability and ameliorates the metabolic syndrome in Zucker diabetic fatty rats. The Journal of Nutrition. 1 Dec 2007;**137**(12):2680-2685

[39] Serino M, Luche E, Gres S, Baylac A, Bergé M, Cenac C, et al. Metabolic adaptation to a high-fat diet is associated with a change in the gut microbiota. Gut. 1 Apr 2012;**61**(4):543-553

[40] Rooks MG, Veiga P, Wardwell-Scott LH, Tickle T, Segata N,

Michaud M, et al. Gut microbiome composition and function in experimental colitis during active disease and treatment-induced remission. The ISME Journal. Jul 2014;**8**(7):1403-1417

[41] Wexler HM. Bacteroides: The good, the bad, and the nitty-gritty. Clinical Microbiology Reviews. Oct 2007;**20**(4):593-621

[42] Dao MC, Everard A, Aron-Wisnewsky J, Sokolovska N, Prifti E, Verger EO, et al. Akkermansia muciniphila and improved metabolic health during a dietary intervention in obesity: Relationship with gut microbiome richness and ecology. Gut. 1 Mar 2016;**65**(3):426-436

[43] Everard A, Lazarevic V, Derrien M, Girard M, Muccioli GG, Neyrinck AM, et al. Responses of gut microbiota and glucose and lipid metabolism to prebiotics in genetic obese and diet-induced leptin-resistant mice. Diabetes. 1 Nov 2011;**60**(11):2775-2786

[44] Anhê FF, Roy D, Pilon G, Dudonné S, Matamoros S, Varin TV, et al. A polyphenol-rich cranberry extract protects from diet-induced obesity, insulin resistance and intestinal inflammation in association with increased Akkermansia spp. population in the gut microbiota of mice. Gut. 1 Jun 2015;**64**(6):872-883

[45] Roopchand DE, Carmody RN, Kuhn P, Moskal K, Rojas-Silva P, Turnbaugh PJ, et al. Dietary polyphenols promote growth of the gut bacterium Akkermansia muciniphila and attenuate high-fat diet–induced metabolic syndrome. Diabetes. 1 Aug 2015;**64**(8):2847-2858

[46] Bruce-Keller AJ, Salbaum JM, Luo M, Blanchard E IV, Taylor CM, Welsh DA, et al. Obese-type gut microbiota induce neurobehavioral changes in the absence of obesity. Biological Psychiatry. 1 Apr 2015;**77**(7):607-615

[47] De Lartigue G, de La Serre CB, Raybould HE. Vagal afferent neurons in high fat diet-induced obesity; intestinal microflora, gut inflammation and cholecystokinin. Physiology & Behavior. 30 Nov 2011;**105**(1):100-105

[48] Collins B, Hoffman J, Martinez K, Grace M, Lila MA, Cockrell C, et al. A polyphenol-rich fraction obtained from table grapes decreases adiposity, insulin resistance and markers of inflammation and impacts gut microbiota in high-fat-fed mice. The Journal of Nutritional Biochemistry. May 2016;**1**(31):150-165

Chapter 3

Considering the Antioxidant Properties of Tea to Improve Human Health

Sabila Nelson

Abstract

One of the highly available drinks consumed across the planet is tea. Scientists know tea for its ability to oppose oxidation, cell death, bacterial growth and replication, inflammation, plus restorative effects of bioengineering due to the possession of several ingredients including catechin types, caffeine, minerals, small amounts of vitamins, and sugars. Scientists believe that tea components are responsible for invigorating the cerebrospinal neural network and regulating wellbeing in human beings through the mutualistic backtracking of infirmities, such as aging, due to the interplay of extraneous harm precipitated by external elements, such as prolonged subjection to harsh heat from the sun which may lead to dermatoheliosis. This scenario later could cause other worrisome conditions, including erythroderma, early aging, anatomical pathology, edema, heat stroke, progression of nonmalignant, and malignancies in various sites. More so, researchers have linked tea use to a reversal in initiation and development of heterometabolic irregularities existing in paltry quantities in reproductive ducts and systems which impacts procreation by proliferating the functionality deficiencies. This chapter will explore and synthesize the literature to advance possible modalities of activity suggested by scientific enlightenment to enhance a better understanding of possible aspects of tea related to improving human health.

Keywords: tea, antioxidants, catechins, polyphenols, health, disease

1. Introduction

Antioxidant properties in tea, exhibit diuretic, anticarcinogenic, and immunity-support, which suppresses the existence and replication of microbes, and prevent inflammation [1], the properties are instrumental in the inhibition and cure of various disorders, including lymphoproliferative conditions, coronary arterial and cerebrovascular maladies, malignancies, hyperglycemia, elevated vital signals, and other nutrition deficiency ailments. The qualification of tea as a healthful drink is premised by nutritionists on its possession of magnificent properties. Tea is utilized by over 3 billion people in more than 160 countries across the globe and is the second-most consumed drink, water being the leading. There is a mass global production of up to three billion kilograms of tea annually, extracted from the leaves, tea buds, or delicate tea stems of the plants of the genus Camellia [1–9].

Research confirms tea (L.) Kuntze is the most widely used plant tea species, with the most important consumers being the Europeans, particularly the British (close to 540 milliliters per day), and a world average of 120 milliliters of tea per day, per person. Consumers have attributed the utilization of tea as a daily libation and folk medicine in China and several Asian states since early times to its subsumption of profuse polyphenols that exert an opposing effect on oxidative tendencies of oxidant elements by synchronizing the signaling pathway of Nrf2, and also vitalizing NF-kB and MAPK pathways [2, 10].

Tea is out there in various forms, each of these tea types has different levels of antioxidants, and analysts have classified them based on the processing methods and fermentation method and skill, geographical, and climatic conditions. The chemical composition of tea changes significantly during the fermentation process, resulting in the production of theaflavins, which add to the usefulness of tea [5, 9, 11]. Consistent with the available literature, the Chinese were the first human beings to consume tea as juice or medicine around 2737 BC. Though the first producers of tea were only China, India, and Kenya, consumption has now spread widely and people from many countries on all continents of the world now cultivate and tea enjoy [5].

2. History and origin of tea

Scholars believe that Shen Nung, the second emperor of China, first recognized tea in 2737 BCE. It was a unique coincidence that the Emperor was a cup of hot water, while resting under a tree shade when a plant leaf blew into the hot water in the cup, he felt a pleasant flavor and continued using tea [12, 13]. According to a narration by Serafini et al. [14], nobody knew much about tea until 1560 when a Portuguese man named Father Jasper de Cruz who was also a Jesuit missionary, encountered and wrote about it.

By as early as 1657, people from England, particularly in London had already realized the importance of tea as a health drink as it was being sold by a few people in the coffee house of Garway. Later on, in 1826, the commercial selling of tea began in seals designed by John Horniman, and later was the introduction of packages in lead-lines. In 1870, twinings of England began a uniform blending of tea.

A few years later, in 1904, Richard Blechynden an Englishman created ice tea. This eventuality preceded the invention of tea bags by Thomas Sullivan in 1908, a then-renowned New York tea importer who could send tea in small silk bags to his clients. It was until 1953 that traders finally introduced the world's first instant tea, which to date became a primary drink throughout Europe, North America, North Africa, and Asia.

3. Sources of oxidants in human bodies

In its entirety, metabolic and respiratory processes in the body initiate the creation of reactive oxygen species (ROS), such as free radicals (O_2^-) from superoxide anions, hydroxyl ions, and peroxides (H_2O_2), including some, which are highly reactive [10] and capable of inducing oxidative ruin to fleshy and corpuscle constituents, such as polypeptides, fats, biomolecules, and nucleic acids, when left unbalanced. Scientists have demonstrated that oxidative stress exacerbates the likelihood of genesis and development of chronic disease conditions once there is an excessive build-up of large aggregates of ROS.

Production of malondialdehyde (MDA) (a major indicator of lipid oxidation), which is a central ingredient of oxidative stress incriminated in unpleasant health effects explains the negative consequences of the action of oxidants on lipids and fats. In his summary of findings, Rasaei [15] recommends a desperate need for interventions, especially the utilization of green tea to augment the body's antioxidant response to be able to counteract oxidative stress and MDA production.

Throughout human lives, people suffer equilibrium disruptions, thanks to human lifestyles; the food, drinking water, coupled with the composition of the air inhaled [16–25], intense physical exercise [26–31], and stress predisposes the superfluous formation of reactive oxygen species in human bodies. Consequently, ROS contains free radicals that steer the emergence of oxidative stress, which vandalizes the anatomy of the human organism, thereby causing a disruption in body functional equilibrium, thus precipitating disorders, such as hardening of the arteries, lymphoproliferative, and/or neurodegenerative upsets (Parkinson's or Alzheimer's disease), or maybe obesity.

A fundamental hunt for straightforwardly available sources of antioxidants perpetuates the steadiness in the middle of creating and eliminating reactive oxygen species, examples of dominant and massively predominant antioxidants are alpha-tocopherol (vitamin E), retinol (vitamin A and vitamin C), and also polyphenolic compounds. The attachment to numerous health- effects, including antioxidant validity to phenolic chemicals is based on findings from rigorous research and has positioned phenols as a vital part of the human diet. Polyphenols can proficiently trap oxidizing peroxide ions, and exterminate lipid radicals, ROS, and hydroxyl radicals.

Polyphenols extracted from plants contribute significantly to decelerating senescent progression and decreased contingency of neurodegenerative conditions related to age, such as Alzheimer's disease, Parkinson's disease, and/or ischemic brain trauma. Some of the natural plant resources, tea, coffee, fruits, vegetables, spices, and herbs are rich sources of antioxidants in the form of flavonoids, which supplement the daily menu, adding up to good health [23].

4. The antioxidant properties of tea

Since the nineteenth century to date, researchers have proclaimed that scientists have competently isolated from tea, more than 500 chemical components, both organic and with different relevancies in maintaining human health [9]. Research findings have further demonstrated and attributed the potential health rewards of drinking tea to the antioxidant nature of tea polyphenols [2]. Over 70 types of tea polyphenols exist (catechins and epicatechin), theaflavins, flavonols and proanthocyanidins, kaempferol, cannabiscetin, and their glycosides [32]. The structural arrangements for the main green tea catechins are shown in **Figure 1**.

Flavonoids from tea exhibit a stronger property that justifies its ability to neutralize ROS/RNS, and, therefore, the antioxidant activity of tea is directly proportional to the amount of flavonols present; the higher, the better. It is equally worth noting that using tea and its components cannot take over the role of standard chemotherapy rather, the beneficial properties of tea, particularly EGCG may be used to complement

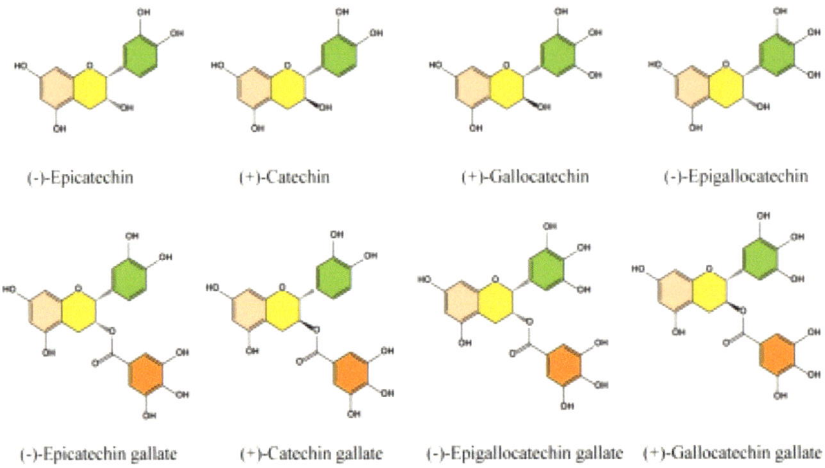

Figure 1.
Structural representation of the main catechins [33].

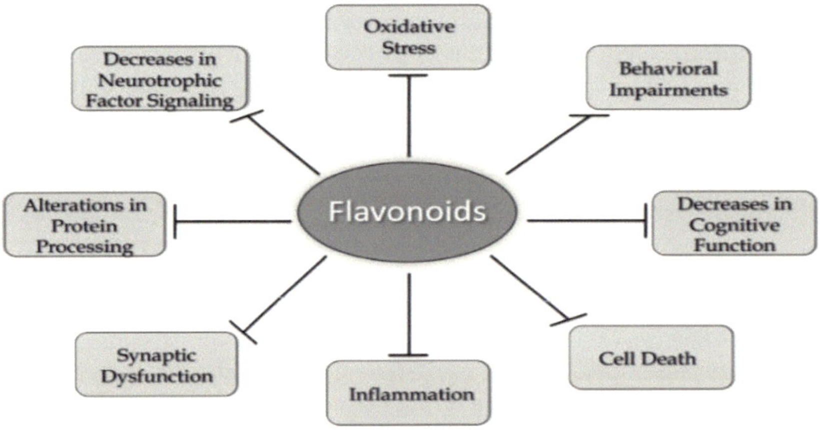

Figure 2.
Showing how Flavonoids alter multiple pathways implicated in brain aging and neurodegenerative diseases [37].

and support the standard anticancer approach [34–36]. **Figure 2** shows the multidimensional role of tea flavonoids.

5. Mechanism of action of antioxidants

Although tea has quite an innumerable number of phenolic chemicals that contribute in isolation or in synergy. EGCG being a major antioxidative player, is instrumental in combating, inflammation, proliferation, and thrombogenesis. It also has a positive impacts on endothelial function.

Experts have surmised tea antioxidants in two ways: in the first place, EGCG breaks the oxidant chain by donating a p-electron on its benzene ring to the available free radical, and by so doing, eliminates the invasive free radicals [12]. In this instance, single electrons tend to the benzene ring, thereby reducing the activity of the hydrogen-oxygen bond in the phenolic hydroxyl group. The hydrogen in phenolic hydroxyl groups participates in the increase and scavenging of free radicals that compete for active oxygen and also terminate the auto-oxidation reaction of the free radicals [10, 38]. Second, phenols remove ROS/RNS to promote the initiation of antioxidants relevant to quenching the formation of cold product chains. Wherefore, improve and protect the antioxidant defense system, chelate available metal ions, strengthen co-oxidants, and/or regulate gene expressions [12, 39].

Yan et al. [10] in their research found that ROS could function at low levels as molecular signals to regulate cellular activities, such as adaptive cellular responses and possible cell growth. Once there is an imbalance between ROS accumulation and the antioxidant process in the body, oxidative stress and damage to cells and tissues become the result, leading to several health anomalies. Further corroborative evidence from research suggests an association between free radicals and the development of diseases, such as arterial hardening, malignancies, emphysema, and others.

Bernatoniene and Kopustinskiene [39] detail how catechins can inhibit the actions of oxidant supporting enzymes, such as NADPH, or modulate the interaction of ligands with receptors like TNF; they are also capable of repressing many pathways related to oxidative stress that is responsible for the processes of inflammation. Catechins are suspect in modulating important responses to pathogenesis-related oxidative stress by facilitating the activities of redox-sensitive transcription factors, enhancement of activated B cells, and activator proteins. The interactive ability of Catechins is possible due to penetrative ability into the membranes of lipid bilayers via adsorption or penetration, hydrogen bonding to protein proline residues, and power to bind to the enzyme ATP-binding sites. **Figure 3** partly explains the role of EGCG in the body.

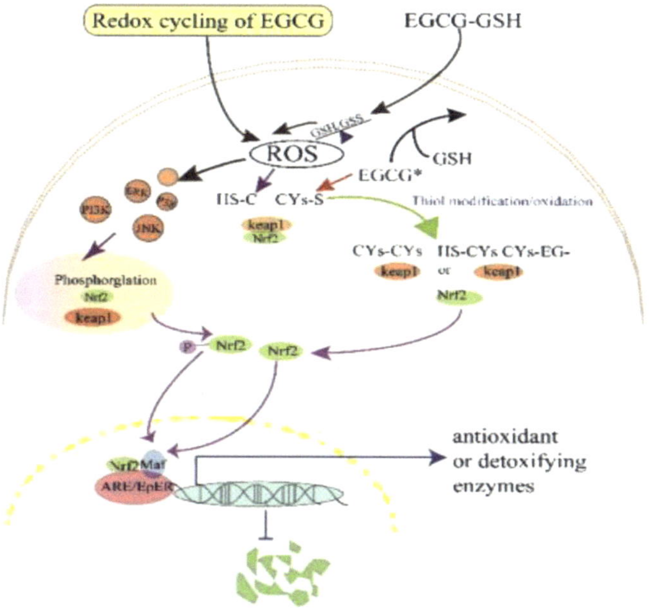

Figure 3.
EGCG induces the up regulation of antioxidant or detoxifying enzymes by Nrf2-ARE signaling [40].

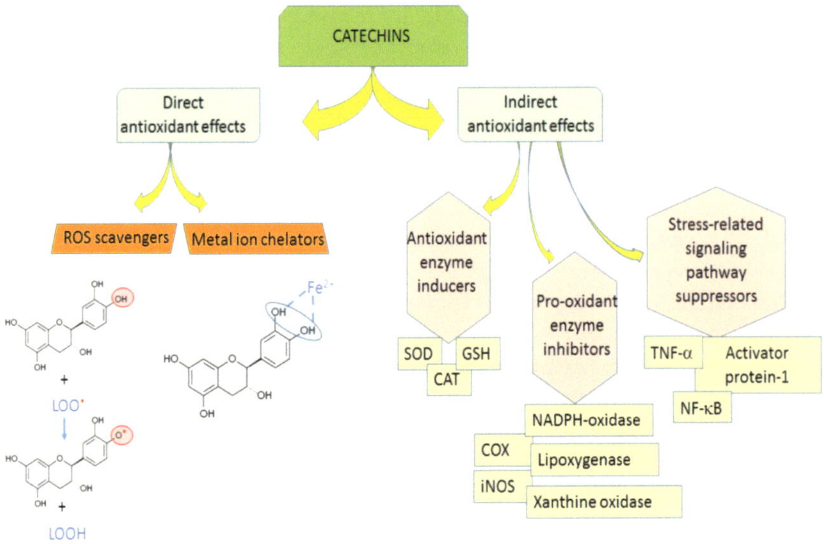

Figure 4.
Antioxidant properties of catechins as adopted from http://www.sciencedirect.com › science

Researchers have also suggested the similar structures and conformational properties of both catechins and transcriptional factors as possible mechanisms for interactions. **Figure 4** illustrates the oxidation mechanism of catechins.

Oz et al. [1] further elucidate how an assortment of reviews has communicated the importance of tea polyphenols as formidable antioxidants in the inactivation of several signaling trails involved in inflammation; down-regulation of Cox-2 and Bcl-2 activities, up-regulation of protective and programmed apoptotic trajectories, and NF-_B mediated pathways of IKK.

6. Health importance of tea antioxidant properties

In this write-up, I will highlight the oxidative impact of tea polyphenols on cancer, cardiovascular conditions, neurodegenerative disorders, diabetes, and their role in boosting fertility in human beings.

6.1 Cancer

The role of EGCG, as an active compound of green tea, is to deter and ameliorate disease courtesy of its antioxidant and anti-inflammatory properties, in conformity the with a validated myriad of study findings. Scientists have proven the effectiveness of this green tea compound in the inhibition of carcinogenesis processes in many types of cancer, though it is still under investigation for effectiveness in other types. Furthermore, catechins are effective in modulating the complexity of chemical processes in the mitochondrion and act in synergy with chemotherapeutic agents to reduce toxicities and anti-carcinogenic outcomes [12, 35, 39, 41]. **Figure 5** shows the spectrum of EGCG action on numerous cancer sites.

Besides hampering the accumulation of ROS in human bodies to prevent cancer, EGCG also blocks the DNA synthesis of cancer cells without interfering with the

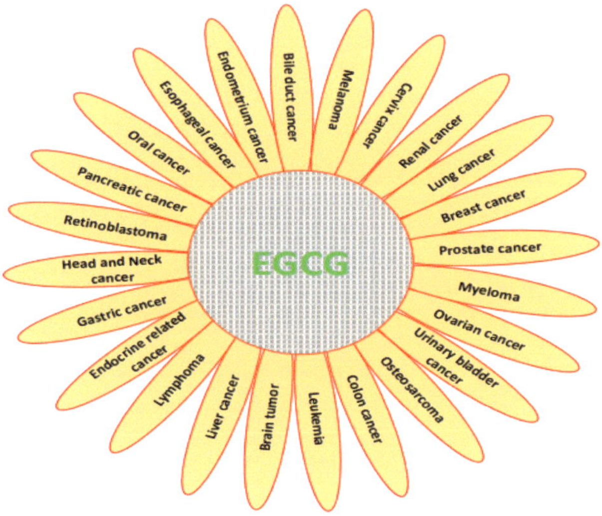

Figure 5.
Role of EGCG in the inhibition of numerous types of cancers [41].

division of normal body cells [10]. In an experiment aimed at establishing the role of EGCG in stimulating hepatocytes in goats, findings revealed efficacy in promoting cell proliferation, improving the integrity of cell membranes, and cell endurance and function under stress from oxidation, [10, 35].

More findings by Niedzwiecki et al. [42] from several other experiments agreed that tea polyphenols, in combination act synergistically to inhibit tumor growth and metastasis, thus efficacious if used against multiple targets and levels of cancer development and progression, and thus, could be a safe and efficacious approach in cancer prevention and therapy.

Given the numerous findings, scientists recommend that medics could use the synergistic competence of tea catechins with anticancer medications to support therapy as well as cancer prevention [43]. Almatroodi et al. [41] further contend that the combined therapy helps to enhance more anti-cancerous activity and reduction of toxicities by the mitigation of the after-effects sometimes witnessed during single chemotherapy use, which though efficacious in the treatment of cancer, and causes adverse side effects, including malaise, hair loss, infection, nausea, and vomiting, appetite complications, mood swings, and changes in physiologic and biochemical processes Tang et al. [44]. See **Figure 6** for illustration.

Further findings from clinical trials as discussed by Musial et al. [35] produced interesting results which portrayed a positive response when Polyphenon E was administered as a supplement, consisting of thriving catechins: EC, EGC, ECG, and EGCG to patients with carcinoma effectiveness. Each capsule contained a decaf EGCG mixture with 200 mg content. During the first phase of the experiment to determine the required dose of EGCG, investigators established a limit of 1200 mg EGCG as a thresh hold for future safety. They also discovered that effective prevention against colorectal adenocarcinoma required consuming ten cups of tea of 150 milliliters each per day.

Other findings from reviews of *in vivo* and *in vitro* studies by Tang et al. [44] recommended the consumption of five cups of tea per day for four weeks to achieve anticancer effectiveness. Also, oral bacteria that could be a causative agent in oral

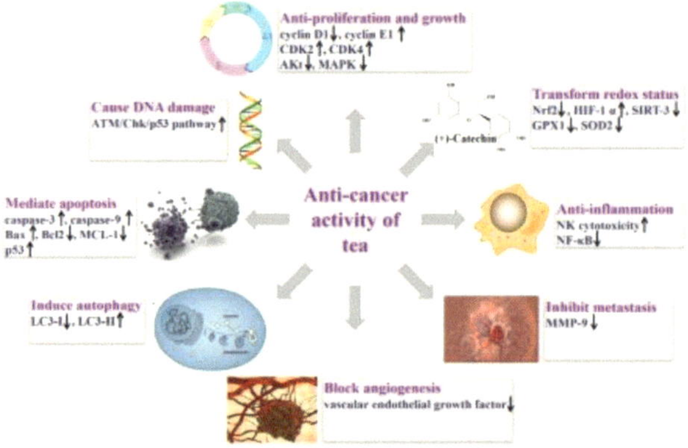

Figure 6.
The most molecular target of tea on targeting cancer [44].

cancer would be neutralized by drinking five cups of infusion tea extracted from two grams of tea daily for six months; this practice also applies to reducing oxidative stress and stopping the initiation of prostate cancer. However, a warning based on findings from an isolated study indicated an increased risk of developing bladder cancer when one consumed five to nine cups of tea per day [35].

6.2 Neurodegenerative diseases

Maher explains neurodegeneration as "any pathological condition which primarily affects neurons," and terms neurodegenerative diseases as an outsized and heterogeneous group of neurological disorders that significantly affect distinct subsets of neurons in specific anatomical locations. Of a wider variety of known neurodegenerative disorders, four are of serious attention, thus Alzheimer's disease (AD), Parkinson's disease (PD), Huntington's disease (HD), and amyotrophic lateral sclerosis.

Researchers believe in an increased likelihood of neurodegenerative conditions due to suspected elevated quantities of ROS in the brain [39, 45], this lowers antioxidant activity in the human brain vis-à-vis other body organs. Accelerated senescence and neurodegeneration are caused by mitochondrial oxidative insults and impaired electron transfer, which often weaken and affect the central nervous system.

Also noted is that oxidative products clog neurons during the aging process. This event calls for the consumption of antioxidant compounds, precisely, catechins that are suspects in the delay and/or stoppage of neurodegenerative processes, and declining brain function [39].

Furthermore, scientific evidence has it that polyphenols can lower the morbidity due to PD and AD by reducing oxidative stress and regulating signaling pathways and metal chelation. Hence, scholars believe that theanine inhibits the glutamate receptors and regulates the extracellular concentration of glutamine, presenting the much-desired neuroprotective effects.

Another possible way that the neuroprotective mode of action by which caffeine and theaflavins contribute is the ability to use their antioxidant properties in antagonizing the adenosine receptor A2AR, respectively. Besides, the element of aroma is a crucial factor affecting tea's sensory quality, with over 600 volatilities identified from the aroma of tea.

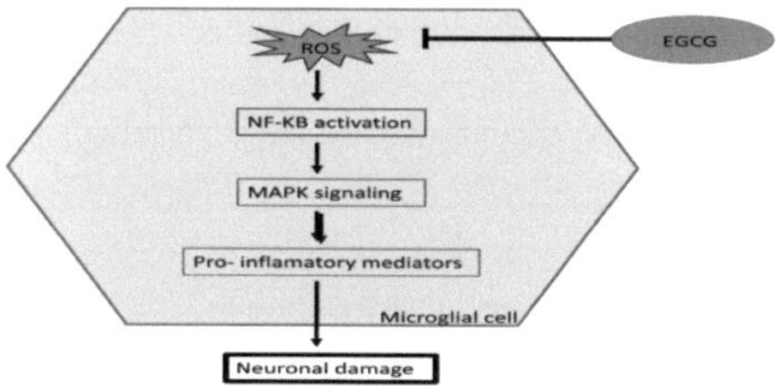

Figure 7.
EGCG inhibition of ROS role in Neuronal damage [45].

Moreover, the legitimately generated tea volatilities from chemical reactions could lessen brain signal dissemination, soothe stress, and experience tranquilizing effects, but the mechanisms have not been well elucidated by experts [3]. From more findings, EGCG suppresses TNF-α, interleukin-1β, interleukin-6, and iNOS, in Aβ energized EOC 13.31, invigorates the extracellular antioxidants certain to nuclear factor 2, as well as the oxygenase1 (HO-1). Ultimately, EGCG also subdues nuclear factor-kB (NF-κB), and prompts the actuation of ROS by the Aβ remedy, as shown in **Figure 7**.

Another central nervous system progressive disorder that has no cure known as paralysis agitans derives its genesis from the destruction of brain cells that produce dopamine. Its impact can be minimized with green tea use as a foremost recommendation by several researchers. The reason for green tea predisposition is the fact that it protects neurons, hence prevents PD, cushions dopamine neurons, provides a shielding effect from ROS, intercepts apoptosis in the brain and CNS, and thus prevents PD [12].

Findings by Vishnoi et al. [12] from an *in vitro* study substantiated the ability of tea to restrain the human acetylcholinesterase with an IC value of 0.03 mg/ml and restrained β-secretase at a test concentration of 0.03 mg/ml by 38%. The study further hypothesized that tea infusion constituted biologically functional truths, conceivably acting in an interactive manner. Physicians could prefer this idea to retard the progression of disease with the presumption that these principles reach the brain.

Scientists think the appliance of EGCG decreases the production of beta-amyloid, a protein that shapes the plaque that obstructs the brains of Alzheimer's casualties and aggravates disease symptoms. Impeding the actions of the enzyme acetylcholinesterase and β-amyloidosis should be the first aspiration for the therapy for Alzheimer's disease [12].

Additional evidence from various studies conducted in Asia and Europe, involving over 290 participants concluded that the outset of PD and AD could amazingly be procrastinated by up to 7.7 years when subjects take between two and three cups of tea on a daily basis [8]. Additional studies have shown the significant roles of tea polyphenols in the treatment of neurodegenerative diseases by protecting the systema nervosum through improvement of learning and memory as in (AD), improvement of nerve redox disparity, and mitochondrial affliction by balancing biological time as in (PD), and lowering of neural vandalism after the cerebral ischemia at an EGCG recommended dose of fifty mg/kg.

Moreover, analysts have reported that consuming an average of 400 mg/kg of green tea polyphenols could lead to an increase in the perceptual-cognitive capacity of patients recovering from chronic cerebral hypoperfusion by scavenging oxygen free radicals, limitation of the creation of lipid peroxides, and mitigating the effect of oxidized DNA, thereby enforcing a neuroprotective function [9].

6.3 Cardiovascular disease

Cardiovascular disease (CVD) is an aggregation of ailments entailing numerous aspects. Amongst those factors are inflammation, cumulative damage done by free radicals, thrombolytic aggregation, and metabolic processes [12]. Other previous studies have highlighted that habitual consumers of green tea were less likely to suffer from diseases of the heart and cardiovascular accidents. Research published by Harvard University further confirms a link between taking tea and wellness; drinking at least one cup of tea daily reduced heart attacks by up to 44%.

Green tea also dramatically raises the antioxidant capacity of the blood, which in effect shields the LDL cholesterol particles from being oxidized, limiting one part of the heart disease pathways. Research findings further entrench that women dying from cardiovascular disease and stroke were lower than 31% for those who consumed five or more cups of tea every day [12].

Oxidative stress has been incriminated as a victim in the progression of various cardiovascular infirmities, including high blood pressure, endothelial dysfunction and hardening of arteries, ischemic heart diseases, cardiomyopathy, cardiac hypertrophy, and congestive heart failure [39].

A summary of findings from over 150 human interventions and animal studies involving more than 35,000 subjects between 1992 and 2017 from across the world by Li et al. Ref. [4] has postulated that tea relaxes muscles facilitating smooth contraction, enhancing endothelial nitric oxide synthase activity, reducing vascular inflammation, inhibiting renin activity, and anti-vascular oxidative stress, thus confirmed that both tea and tea metabolites have anti-hypertensive effects in *ex vivo* tissue and *in vitro* cell culture studies, although some controversial reports existed [39].

Correspondingly, wrap-up evidence from a plethora of studies by Serafini et al. [14] deduced that taking a capsule containing theaflavin-enriched GTE (375 mg) daily with two cups of GT, containing about 250 mg of total catechins could provide tea flavan-3-ols enough to control CVDs by up to 10 mg/dL [0.25 mmol/L] of LDL.

6.4 Diabetes

Diabetes is a serious global, long-term condition with a major impact on the lives and well-being of individuals, families, and societies worldwide [46, 47]. Diabetes is an amalgam of metabolic conditions that cause high blood sugar and could be a result of autoimmune and hereditary defects. High blood glucose is either because of impaired insulin production, low cellular sensitivity to insulin, or a combination of the two factors [48].

Diabetes is one of the top 10 causes of death among grownups, causing an estimated four million deaths globally in 2017. During the same year, 2017, global health expenditure on diabetes soared to a high USD 727 billion [49] Diabetes is into three categories; T1D, T2D, and GDM [48].

It may not be feasible to prevent T1D but is treatable by health professionals with insulin supplementation, whereas T2D can both be averted, and/or reversed by altering diet and management of lifestyle factors [46]. T2D is a heterogeneous disorder, characterized by the resistance of glucose and lipid metabolism in peripheral tissues to the biological activity of insulin, and inadequate secretion of insulin by pancreatic β cells [12], the loss of functional β-cell mass plays a central role in the deterioration of blood glucose control [50], inherited and/or acquired deficiencies in insulin secretion and/or by decreased responsiveness of the organs to secrete insulin also called insulin resistance culminates into increased blood glucose, this in turn can damage many of the body's systems, including blood vessels and nerves [51].

Diabetes has high morbidity and mortality, attributed to its complications, such as diabetic nephropathy, diabetic cardiovascular complications, diabetic neuropathy, diabetic retinopathy, and diabetic hepatopathy [52]. An aggregate of findings by Imran et al. [53] from several experiments using rats to determine the effects of theaflavins and thearugibin drink on blood glucose levels indicated a reduction in cholesterol, LDL, and triglyceride levels of experimental rats in all studies with a significant increase in HDL. In this context, theaflavins-based drink imparted maximum reduction in cholesterol, the highest glucose decline, and maximum insulin increase in all studies as compared to other nutraceutical drinks.

Functional drinks can be useful for combating lifestyle-related maladies with special reference to hypercholesterolemia and hyperglycemia. What's more, Li et al. [4] reported consequential therapeutic qualities of tea on hypertensive diabetic patients where diabetics who took green tea infusions after meals, three times daily for a period of four weeks, had their blood pressure reduced significantly. In a short time of 15 days, both the SBP and DBP had reduced significantly by 4.6 mmHg and 3.6 mmHg, respectively.

A similar case-control study meant to determine the effects of green tea extracts involved diabetic Japanese adults and a control group who were healthy and revealed a noticeable drop in sugar levels with the continued use of the tea extract.

In consensus with earlier studies, further evidence was generated with findings from more clinical trials communicating the effectiveness of tea intervention on diabetics and patients with related complications [54], and the important biologic activities of green tea in anti-diabetic makeup [9]. See **Figure 8**.

Contemporaneous studies have also imputed the anti-diabetic effect of green tea mainly in the following mechanisms; the potential to reduce insulin resistance by

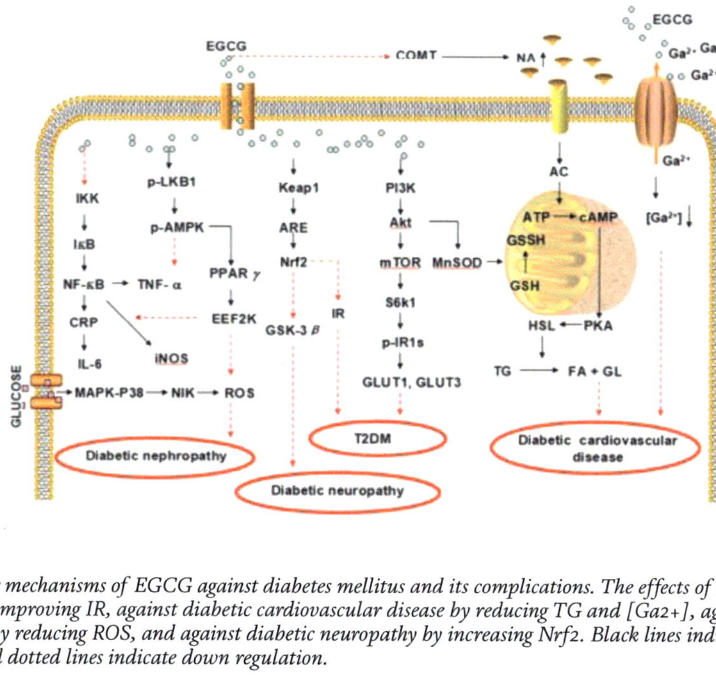

Figure 8.
The molecular mechanisms of EGCG against diabetes mellitus and its complications. The effects of ECG against T2D show by improving IR, against diabetic cardiovascular disease by reducing TG and [Ga2+], against diabetic nephropathy by reducing ROS, and against diabetic neuropathy by increasing Nrf2. Black lines indicate up regulation, red dotted lines indicate down regulation.

increasing the absorption of glucose by adipocytes and their ability to bind to insulin [51, 54], the power to enhance glucose metabolism by triggering an increase in glycogen content in the liver, change of the activity of key enzymes in glucose metabolism [43, 46], ameliorating insulin secretion, and amortizing diabetic complications [9].

In another study, investigators administered 500 mg/kg of green tea polyphenols to normal rats during an experiment. By the lapse of sixty minutes, the glucose tolerance had raised notably. A significant reduction in blood sugar in alloxan diabetic rats at specified doses, and for a given period of time justified the significance role that tea plays in improving glycolysis and lipogenesis [12].

Carotenoids in green tea play both a functional role as pro-vitamin A in the visual pathway and a structural role as macular pigments further upholding the antioxidant potency of tea in the prevention and treatment of T2DM [55]. Meanwhile, transpiring corroboration portrays the capacity of phenols to aid the secretion of intestinal L-cells and could be useful in the improvement of glycolysis and homeostasis [49].

Quercetin, another strong antioxidant component in tea has the potential to reduce insulin resistance and decrease inflammation by improving the expression of glucose transporters GLUT4 [8].

Tang et al. [44] tabled findings from several clinical trials with optimism in managing T2DM, in relation to ameliorating insulin resistance and hyperglycemia in humans. The findings advance a postulation that drinking black tea could significantly reduce the glycated hemoglobin levels (HbA1c) and ameliorated the likelihood of ailment due to T2D. Moreover, the same findings confirm that T2D aggravated by diets rich in high fat could as well be contained by regularly taking green tea.

6.5 Infertility

Human infertility is a global concern and already affects one in six couples worldwide [56], research approximates that between 15 and 30% of couples are struggling to conceive [33]. Male factors contribute to 20–50% of the cases, making infertility a controversial problem across the globe, some of the factors point to several anatomical discrepancies, including but not limited to obstructions in seminal tubes, neurological anomalies, aging, and urinary tract infections, these affect spermatogenesis and weakening the sperm function.

It is also worth noting that an interplay of several environmental factors exist that reduce semen quality, hence, infertility, such as tobacco use, excessive consumption of alcohol, exposure of testis to higher temperatures, dietary inadequacies, oxidative stress, and exposure to industrial chemicals, pesticides, and radiation. An understanding of cell biology correlates with the assumption that increased levels of ROS lead to a lower antioxidant response, which is not healthy for sperm production and quality [33, 56, 57] as shown in **Figure 9**.

A synopsis of evidence by Zhang et al. [40] suggests that the secondary metabolite in green tea (EGCG) portrays diverse physiologic activities, including antioxidant, antitumor, and antiviral activities, single or a conglomerate of which could be a recipe for infertility. Further to this, investigators found that fertility in human beings is supported by EGCG through the mitigation of the impacts of excessive ROS on sperm and oocyte cells, cell death, hyperactivation of enzymes on the ERK, and signal regulating proteins operating outside cells.

According to Rahman et al. [33, 45], the high presence of antioxidants in EGCG, can reduce ROS and improve gamete quality in both males and females, at low concentrations, and that supplementation with EGCG in males can considerably increase

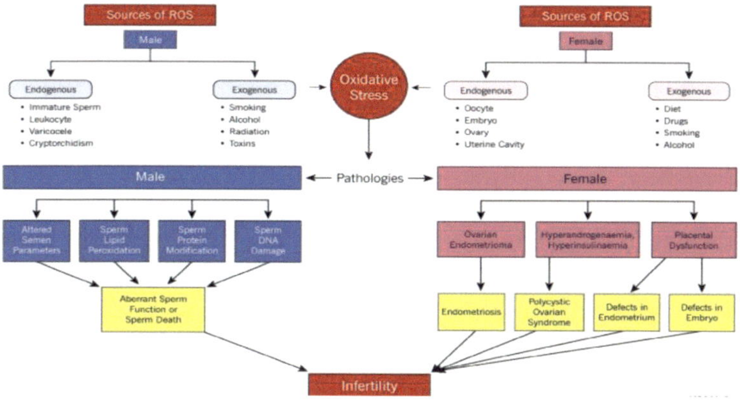

Figure 9.
Sources of oxidative stress and their impact on reproduction and fertility [57].

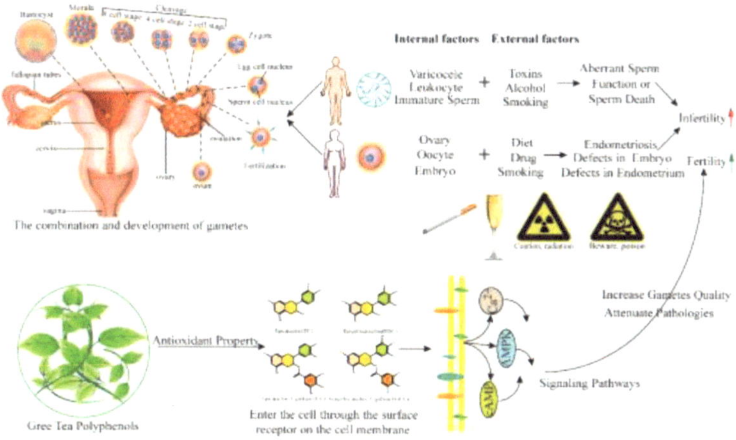

Figure 10.
The action of green tea polyphenols on major fertility reducing factors [33].

sperm concentration, motility, fertility rate, morphology, and viability, and reduce DNA damage. It is also capable of enhancing the quality of oocytes and embryos, hence, increasing the rates of fertilization and clinical pregnancy in female beings. Consistently, using green tea has an inverse relationship with the risk of ovarian cancer, which is a factor in female infertility; a further illustration is shown in **Figure 10**.

7. Conclusion

Over the years, there has been global consumption of tea, both for recreational and medicinal purposes. This has been attributed to the demonstrated health benefits, mainly, its antioxidant properties are instrumental in suppressing the initiation, onset, and progression of metabolic disorders, different types of malignancies, degenerative diseases, infertility complications dermatological problems, respiratory infections insulin resistance, and osteoporosis. Although some studies have provided controversial results about the safety of tea and its products in excess, scientists could not provide an independent confirmation but may be a subject for future research, in comparison with the overwhelming evidence from numerous studies on the benefits and safety of tea and its constituent components. Areas of further exploration should interest in the sustainable bioavailability of tea and its products for intended purposes, more findings on the mechanism of action by tea and its products in the improvement of health, and further need to study the interactive capabilities with other medications and supplements. By and large, the consumption of tea for recreation and medicinal reasons hitherto remains safe and recommended.

Acknowledgements

I want to sincerely thank IntechOpen Team for the world-class publication and for providing me the opportunity to have my work published. Ms Marica Novakovic, has particularly been very helpful, thank you so much.

Conflict of interest

The author declares no conflict of interest.

Acronyms

ACC	acetyl-CoA carboxylase
AMD	adjusted mean difference
BMI	body mass index
CAT	*catalase* EC-epicatechin
CI	confidence interval
COX	*cyclooxygenase*
CRP	reactive protein
DBP	diastolic blood pressure
ECG	epicatechin-3-gallate
EGC	epigallocatechin
EGCG	epigallocatechin-3-gallate
FAS/FASN	fatty acid synthase
FAs	fatty acids
GCG	gallocatechin gallate
GrTPs	green tea polyphenols
GSH	*glutathione peroxidase*
GST	glutathione S-transferase
GT	green tea
GTE	green tea extract
HSL	hormone-sensitive lipase
IKK	Inhibitory Kappa B Kinase complex
iNOS	*inducible nitric oxide synthase*
LPS	lipopolysaccharide
LXR	liver X receptor
LDL	low-density lipoprotein

MAPK	mitogen-activated protein kinase
MDA	malondialdehyde
MetS	metabolic syndrome
MS	multiple sclerosis
NADPH-oxidase	nicotinamide adenine dinucleotide phosphate oxidase
NAFLD	non-alcoholic fatty liver disease
NF-_B	nuclear factor kappa-light-chain-enhancer of activated B cells
NF-kB	nuclear factor kappa light chain enhancer of activated B cells
Nrf2	nuclear factor erythroid-2 related factor
Ors	odds ratios
PGC-1α	peroxisome proliferator-activated receptor-γ coactivator-1α
PPAR	peroxisome proliferation-activated receptor
RCT	randomized controlled trial
ROS	reactive oxygen species
SBP	systolic blood pressure
SCD	stearoyl-CoA desaturase
SIRT	sirtuin
SOD	superoxide dismutase
SREBP	sterol regulatory element-binding proteins
TC	total cholesterol
Tcf7l2	transcription factor 7-like 2
TFA	total abdominal fat area
TGs	triglycerides
TNF	tumor necrosis factor
UA	uric acid
VEGF	vascular endothelial growth factor
VFA	visceral fat area
WC	waist circumference
WMD	weighted mean difference

Author details

Sabila Nelson
Independent Scientist, Mbale, Uganda

*Address all correspondence to: sabila840@gmail.com

References

[1] Oz HS. Chronic inflammatory diseases and green tea polyphenols. Nutrients. 2017;**9**(6):561

[2] Truong VL, Jeong WS. Cellular defensive mechanisms of tea polyphenols: Structure-activity relationship. International Journal of Molecular Sciences. 2021;**22**(17):9109

[3] Chen SQ, Wang ZS, Ma YX, Zhang W, Lu JL, Liang YR, et al. Neuroprotective effects and mechanisms of tea bioactive components in neurodegenerative diseases. Molecules. 2018;**23**(3):512

[4] Li D, Wang R, Huang J, Cai Q, Yang CS, Wan X, et al. Effects and mechanisms of tea regulating blood pressure: Evidences and promises. Nutrients. 2019;**11**(5):1115

[5] Malar DS, Prasanth MI, Brimson JM, Sharika R, Sivamaruthi BS, Chaiyasut C, et al. Neuroprotective properties of green tea (*Camellia sinensis*) in Parkinson's disease: A review. Molecules. 2020;**25**(17):3926

[6] Vyas T, Nagi R, Bhatia A, Bains SK. Therapeutic effects of green tea as an antioxidant on oral health: A review. Journal of Family Medicine and Primary Care. 2021;**10**(11):3998-4001

[7] Moldoveanu SC, Oden R. Antioxidant character and levels of polyphenols in several tea samples. ACS Omega. 2021;**6**(15):9982-9988

[8] Pérez-Torres I, Castrejón-Téllez V, SotoME,Rubio-RuizME,Manzano-PechL, &Guarner-Lans, V. Oxidative stress, plant natural antioxidants, and obesity. International Journal of Molecular Sciences. 2021;**22**(4):1786

[9] Zhao T, Li C, Wang S, Song X. Green tea (*Camellia sinensis*): A review of its phytochemistry, pharmacology, and toxicology. Molecules. 2022;**27**(12):3909

[10] Yan Z, Zhong Y, Duan Y, Chen Q, Li F. Antioxidant mechanism of tea polyphenols and its impact on health benefits. Animal Nutrition (Zhongguoxu mu shouyixuehui). 2020;**6**(2):115-123

[11] Tong T, Liu Y-J, Kang J, Zhang C-M, Kang S-G. Antioxidant activity and main chemical components of a novel fermented tea. Molecules. 2019;**24**(16):2917

[12] Vishnoi H, Bodla RB, Kant R, Bodla RB. Green tea (*Camellia sinensis*) and its antioxidant property: A review. International Journal of Pharmaceutical Sciences and Research. 2018;**9**(5):1723-1736

[13] Wambulwa MC, Meegahakumbura MK, Kamunya S, Wachira FN. From the wild to the cup: Tracking footprints of the tea species in time and space. Frontiers Nutrition. 6 Aug 2021;**8**:706770. DOI: 10.3389/fnut.2021.706770. PMID: 34422884; PMCID: PMC8377202

[14] Serafini M, Del Rio D, Yao DN, Bettuzzi S, Peluso I. Health benefits of tea. In: Herbal Medicine: Biomolecular and Clinical Aspects. 2nd ed. Boca Raton (FL): CRC Press/Taylor & Francis; 2011

[15] Rasaei N, Asbaghi O, Samadi M, Setayesh L, Bagheri R, Gholami F, et al. Effect of green tea supplementation on antioxidant status in adults: A systematic review and meta-analysis of randomized clinical trials. Antioxidants. 2021;**10**(11):1731

[16] Chen L, Mo H, Zhao L, Gao W, Wang S, Cromie MM, et al. Therapeutic

properties of green tea against environmental insults. The Journal of Nutrition Biochemistry. Feb 2017;**40**:1-13. DOI: 10.1016/j.jnutbio.2016.05.005. Epub 2016 May 27. PMID: 27723473; PMCID: PMC5124528

[17] Duracova M, Klimentova J, Fucikova A, Dresler J. Proteomic methods of detection and quantification of protein toxins. Toxins. 2018;**10**(3):99

[18] Navarro M, McClane B, Uzal F. Mechanisms of action and cell death associated with clostridium perfringens toxins. Toxins. 2018;**10**(5):212

[19] Nelson S, David N, Stephen K, Christopher D. Risk Factors for Esophageal Cancer among Adults Aged 40 Years and Above in Sebei Region, Eastern Uganda. 2018

[20] Arregui L, Ayala M, Gómez-Gil X, Gutiérrez-Soto G, Hernández-Luna CE, et al. Laccases: Structure, function, and potential application in water bioremediation. Microbial Cell Factories. 2019;**18**(1):200

[21] Grootveld M, Percival BC, Leenders J, Wilson PB. Potential adverse public health effects afforded by the ingestion of dietary lipid oxidation product toxins: Significance of fried food sources. Nutrients. 2020;**12**(4):974

[22] Bojková B, Winklewski PJ, Wszedybyl-Winklewska M. Dietary fat and cancer-which is good, which is bad, and the body of evidence. International Journal of Molecular Sciences. 2020;**21**(11):4114

[23] Jakubczyk K, Kałduńska J, Kochman J, Janda K. Chemical profile and antioxidant activity of the Kombucha beverage derived from white, green, black and red tea. Antioxidants. 2020;**9**(5):447

[24] Serafini MM, Catanzaro M, Fagiani F, Simoni E, Caporaso R, Dacrema M, et al. Modulation of Keap1/Nrf2/ARE signaling pathway by curcuma-and garlic-derived hybrids. Frontiers in Pharmacology. 2020;**10**:1597

[25] Yan LJ, Allen DC. Cadmium-induced kidney injury: Oxidative damage as a unifying mechanism. Biomolecules. 2021;**11**(11):1575

[26] Cavalcante PAM, Gregnani MF, Henrique JS, et al. Aerobic but not resistance exercise can induce inflammatory pathways via toll-like 2 and 4: A systematic review. Sports Medicine. 2017;**3**:42

[27] Kim JS, Lee YH, Chang YU, et al. PPARγ regulates inflammatory reaction by inhibiting the MAPK/NF-κB pathway in C2C12 skeletal muscle cells. Journal of Physiology and Biochemistry. 2017;**73**:49-57

[28] Magherini F, Fiaschi T, Marzocchini R, Mannelli M, Gamberi T, Modesti PA, et al. Oxidative stress in exercise training: The involvement of inflammation and peripheral signals. Free Radical Research. 2019;**53**(11-12):1155-1165

[29] Aicale R, Tarantino D, Maffulli N. Overuse injuries in sport: A comprehensive overview. Journal of Orthopaedic Surgery and Research. 2018;**13**:309

[30] Kruk J, Kotarska K, Aboul-Enein BH. Physical exercise and catecholamines response: Benefits and health risk: Possible mechanisms. Free Radical Research. 2020;**54**(2-3):105-125

[31] Flockhart M, Nilsson LC, Tais S, Ekblom B, Apró W, Larsen FJ. Excessive exercise training causes mitochondrial functional impairment and decreases glucose tolerance in

healthy volunteers. Cell Metabolism. 2021;**33**(5):957-970

[32] Samanta S. Potential bioactive components and health promotional benefits of tea (*Camellia sinensis*). Journal of the American Nutrition Association. 2022;**41**(1):65-93

[33] Rahman SU, Huang Y, Zhu L, Feng S, Khan IM, Wu J, et al. Therapeutic role of green tea polyphenols in improving fertility: A review. Nutrients. 2018;**10**(7):834

[34] Prasanth MI, Sivamaruthi BS, Chaiyasut C, Tencomnao T. A review of the role of green tea (*Camellia sinensis*) in antiphotoaging, stress resistance, neuroprotection, and autophagy. Nutrients. 2019;**11**(2):474

[35] Musial C, Kuban-Jankowska A, Gorska-Ponikowska M. Beneficial properties of green tea catechins. International Journal of Molecular Sciences. 2020;**21**(5):1744

[36] Peluso I, Serafini M. Antioxidants from black and green tea: From dietary modulation of oxidative stress to pharmacological mechanisms. British Journal of Pharmacology. Jun 2017;**174**(11):1195-1208. DOI: 10.1111/bph.13649. Epub 2016 Nov 12. PMID: 27747873; PMCID: PMC5429329

[37] Maher P. The potential of flavonoids for the treatment of neurodegenerative diseases. International Journal of Molecular Sciences. 2019;**20**(12):3056

[38] Zhou B, Ma B, Ma C, Xu C, Wang J, Wang Z, et al. Classification of Pu-erh ripened teas and their differences in chemical constituents and antioxidant capacity. LWT. 2022;**153**(2022):112370

[39] Bernatoniene J, Kopustinskiene DM. The role of catechins in cellular responses to oxidative stress. Molecules. 2018;**23**(4):965

[40] Zhang Y, Lin H, Liu C, Huang J, Liu Z. A review for physiological activities of EGCG and the role in improving fertility in humans/mammals. Biomedicine & Pharmacotherapy, Volume. 2020;**127**:110186

[41] Almatroodi SA, Almatroudi A, Khan AA, Alhumaydhi FA, Alsahli MA, Rahmani AH. Potential therapeutic targets of Epigallocatechin Gallate (EGCG), the most abundant catechin in green tea, and its role in the therapy of various types of cancer. Molecules. 2020;**25**:3146

[42] Niedzwiecki A, Roomi MW, Kalinovsky T, Rath M. Anticancer efficacy of polyphenols and their combinations. Nutrients. 2016;**8**(9):552

[43] Kochman J, Jakubczyk K, Antoniewicz J, Mruk H, Janda K. Health benefits and chemical composition of matcha green tea: A review. Molecules. 2020;**26**(1):85

[44] Tang GY, Meng X, Gan RY, Zhao CN, Liu Q, Feng YB, et al. Health functions and related molecular mechanisms of tea components: An update review. International Journal of Molecular Sciences. 2019;**20**(24):6196

[45] LIczbiński P, Bukowska B. Tea and coffee polyphenols and their biological properties based on the latest in vitro investigations. Industrial Crops and Products. 2022;**175**:114265

[46] Khan N, Mukhtar H. Tea polyphenols in promotion of human health. Nutrients. 2018;**11**(1):39

[47] Nguyen TT, Ta QTH, Nguyen TKO, Nguyen TTD, Van Giau V. Type 3 diabetes and its role implications in Alzheimer's

disease. International Journal of Molecular Sciences. 2020;**21**(9):3165

[48] Winiarska-Mieczan A, Tomaszewska E, Jachimowicz K. Antioxidant, anti-inflammatory, and immunomodulatory properties of tea-the positive impact of tea consumption on patients with autoimmune diabetes. Nutrients. 2021;**13**(11):3972

[49] Premlata RB, Vimlesh SC. Role of Vidangadi Kwatha in Madhumeha (Diabetes Mellitus Type II). Archives of Clinical and Medical Case Reports. 2021;**5**(5):629-633

[50] Saeedi P, Petersohn I, Salpea P, Malanda, B, Karuranga S, Unwin N, Williams Rhys et al. Global and regional diabetes prevalence estimates for 2019 and projections for 2030 and 2045, Results from the International Diabetes Federation Diabetes Atlas , Diabetes Research and Clinical Practice. 2019;157:107843

[51] Takemoto M, Takemoto H. Synthesis of theaflavins and their functions. Molecules. 2018;**23**(4):918

[52] Wang Y, Alkhalidy H, Liu D. The emerging role of polyphenols in the management of Type 2 diabetes. Molecules. 2021;**26**(3):703

[53] Imran A, Butt MS, Arshad MS, et al. Exploring the potential of black tea based flavonoids against hyperlipidemia related disorders. Lipids in Health and Disease. 2018;**17**:57

[54] Meng J-M, Cao S-Y, Wei X-L, Gan R-Y, Wang Y-F, Cai S-X, et al. Effects and mechanisms of tea for the prevention and management of diabetes mellitus and diabetic complications: An updated review. Antioxidants. 2019;**8**(6):170

[55] Roohbakhsh A, Karimi G, Iranshahi M. Carotenoids in the treatment of diabetes mellitus and its complications: A mechanistic review. Biomedicine & Pharmacotherapy. 2017;**91**:31-42

[56] Martin-Hidalgo B, Batista O, Alves. Antioxidants and male fertility: From molecular studies to clinical evidence. Antioxidants. 2019;**8**(4):89

[57] Roychoudhury S, Agarwal A, Virk G, Cho CL. Potential role of green tea catechins in the management of oxidative stress-associated infertility. Reproductive Biomedicine Online. 2017;**34**(5):487-498

Chapter 4

Green Tea with Its Active Compound EGCG for Acute Ischemic Stroke Treatment

Abdulloh Machin and Shafira Putri Widiawan

Abstract

The current standard of treatment for acute ischemic stroke is thrombolysis. However, only less than 2% of the world undergo thrombolysis. Recent studies have shown that Citicholin, one of the popular neuroprotectants, is less effective as stroke therapy, so it is necessary to develop a new approach to protective therapy for ischemic stroke patients. Green tea (Camellia sinensis) is the most consumed beverage in the world and is a source of polyphenols known as catechins, including epigallocatechin-3-gallate (EGCG), which is 63% of total catechins. Many studies explain that green tea consumption will decrease stroke risk, but not many studies explain its benefit in treating acute stroke. This chapter will discuss the benefit of green tea in acute stroke. C. sinensis with the active ingredient EGCG inhibits neuronal cell death through apoptosis and necroptosis in acute ischemic stroke as in the Rattus norvegicus model of Middle Cerebral Artery Occlusion (MCAO), it also can decrease necroptosis and increase M2 type microglia. The study on the benefit of green tea should be conducted in the clinical setting to know the benefit of green tea in acute ischemic stroke. Its potential benefit can be an adjunct treatment for acute ischemic stroke besides standard treatment.

Keywords: green tea, Camellia sinensis, EGCG, acute stroke, stroke treatment

1. Introduction

According to WHO, stroke is a focal or global neurological deficit that more than 24 hours or dies before 24 hours, caused by vascular disorders in the brain [1–3]. There are three types of strokes: ischemic stroke, intracerebral hemorrhage, and spontaneous subarachnoid hemorrhage. Ischemic stroke is the most common type in about 70–80% of stroke cases [4]. Stroke is the second leading cause of death in the world and caused the death of 5.7 million people in 2005 [2, 5, 6]. Around 69% of stroke cases occur in low- and middle-income countries, about 71% of the 5.9 million stroke cases [7–9]. Most stroke patients will have a residual disability, although about 50–70% return to functional independence [10]. Based on this, it is necessary to understand the pathogenesis so that an acute ischemic stroke therapy approach can be carried out [6, 11].

The current standard of treatment for acute ischemic stroke is thrombolysis. However, only 2–8.5% of stroke patients can undergo thrombolysis in America, and less than 2% in the world undergo thrombolysis [2, 3, 12]. During 1995–2015, 430 candidates for stroke therapy were divided into two categories, namely thrombolytic agents and neuroprotectants [13–15]. One of the popular neuroprotectants used in stroke therapy is Citicholin. However, recent studies have shown that Citicholin is less effective as stroke therapy, so it is necessary to develop a new approach to protective therapy for ischemic stroke patients [16–20].

Acute stroke is caused by decrease blood flow, a decrease in the amount of Adenosine triphosphate (ATP). This event will cause lactic acidosis and loss of ion homeostasis in neuronal cells [21]. In addition, disruption of ion homeostasis will cause high levels of calcium and Adenosine diphosphate (ADP) in the cells, which will stimulate mitochondrial reactive oxygen species (ROS) and other sources of free radicals [22–24].

Green tea (*C. sinensis*) is the most consumed beverage in the world and is a source of polyphenols known as catechins, including epigallocatechin-3-gallate (EGCG), which is 63% of total catechins [25–31]. A meta-analysis showed that individuals who consumed 3 cups a day had a 21% lower risk of stroke than those who consumed <1 cup of tea daily [26, 32]. Many studies in animal models have shown that administering EGCG to ischemia–reperfusion brain tissue will reduce the expansion of ischemia [33, 34]. EGCG is also a potent free radical scavenger and can protect neuronal cells from oxidative damage induced by prooxidants [35]. Green tea with the active ingredient EGCG has a role in preventing neuronal cell death in ischemic conditions by inhibiting oxidative stress and improving mitochondrial function [25, 27, 28, 36]. Many studies explain that green tea consumption will decrease stroke risk, but not many studies explain the benefit of green tea in the treatment of acute stroke. This chapter will discuss the benefit of green tea in acute stroke [33, 37].

2. Pathophysiology of ischemic stroke

There is a decrease in blood supply which causes a reduction in the amount of ATP in acute ischemic stroke. This condition leads to anaerobic metabolism with the result of lactic acid. The decrease in blood flow also causes an imbalance in ion homeostasis in neuronal cells and leads ischemic cascade that will be followed by multimodal and multicellular mechanisms that cause neuronal cell death [6, 21].

Severe cerebral ischemia also causes loss of energy stores, ion imbalance, the release of excitatory neurotransmitters, and inhibition of glutamate re-uptake [6, 38]. In addition, glutamate will bind to NMDA and AMPA receptors which will cause calcium influx [1, 39]. This calcium overload will cause the stimulation of phospholipases and proteases that will degrade membranes and proteins [38]. Glutamate receptors also cause sodium and water influx and cause cell swelling, edema, and shrinkage of the extracellular space [6, 40]. In addition, the influx of excessive calcium causes the activation of catabolic processes that will activate proteases, lipases, and nucleases [1, 6, 39].

High calcium, sodium, and ADP levels in ischemic cells will stimulate the production of oxygen radicals in the mitochondria, accompanied by the production of free radicals from other sources such as prostaglandins and the degradation of hypoxanthine [39, 41]. These reactive oxygen species (ROS) will damage membrane lipids, proteins, nucleic acids, and carbohydrates [23, 42, 43]. Furthermore, these

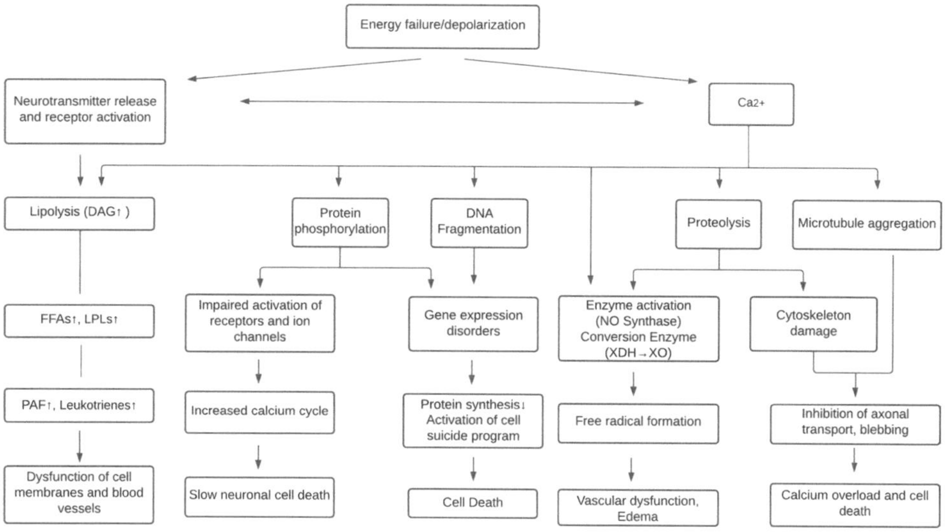

Figure 1.
Ischemic cascade in stroke [47].

ROS are toxic because their basal levels are related to the upregulation of antioxidant enzymes such as SOD, catalase, and glutathione and the scavenger mechanism (α-tocopherol, vitamin C), which is too slow to respond to the production of these ROS [6, 39]. Along with the above mechanism, there will also be a process known as Cortical spreading depression (CSD) which is the depolarization of neurons and glial cells that will spread to surrounding cells at a speed of 2–6 mm/minute [44]. CSD is characterized by an almost complete breakdown of the ion gradient associated with volume shrinkage, loss of electrical activity, swelling of neuron cells, and distortion of dendrites [43, 45]. CSD occurs when the extracellular K+ level exceeds a critical threshold [43]. This CSD wave in ischemic conditions will reach the peri-ischemic area and expand the infarct area (**Figure 1**) [6, 46, 47].

3. Ischemic stroke and oxidative stress

Uncontrolled oxidative stress, an imbalance between pro-oxidant and antioxidant levels that support pro-oxidants, can cause cell, tissue, and organ injury [22]. High Reactive Oxygen Species (ROS) are known to cause direct damage to lipids [43, 48]. The primary sources of endogenous ROS production are mitochondria, plasma membranes, endoplasmic reticulum, and peroxisomes through various mechanisms, including enzymatic reactions and/or autoxidation of several compounds, such as catecholamines and hydroquinones. In addition, different exogenous stimuli, such as ionizing radiation, ultraviolet light, tobacco smoke, pathogenic infections, environmental toxins, and exposure to herbicides/insecticides, are sources of ROS production in vivo [49].

The two most common ROS affecting lipids are hydroxyl radicals (HO) and hydroperoxyl (HO_2). The hydroxyl radical (HO) is a small, active, water-soluble, and chemically reactive oxygen species. This short-lived molecule can be produced from O_2 in cellular metabolism under various stress conditions [48, 50]. These radicals can be neutralized or even attack other biomolecules in the cell. Hydroxyl radicals cause oxidative damage to cells because they are not determined by how much they attack biomolecules and are involved in cellular disorders such as neurodegeneration, cardiovascular disease, and cancer. It is generally assumed that HO in biological systems is formed through a redox reaction by the Fenton reaction; in this reaction, iron (Fe^{2+}) reacts with hydrogen peroxide (H_2O_2), and the Haber–Weiss reaction results in the production of Fe^{2+} when superoxide reacts with ferrous iron (Fe^{3+}). In addition to the iron redox cycle described above, several other transition metals, including Cu, Ni, and Co, can be responsible for forming HO in living cells [22, 48].

Heme oxygenase (HO) is a crucial enzyme of Heme metabolism. The HO-1 isoform is expressed mainly in vascular structures but is very low in normal CNS and can be induced after brain tissue injury. HO-1 is strongly induced after ischemia and will be overexpressed and play a protective role against ischemia after permanent vascular occlusion [6, 51–55].

An initial study to determine the role of HO-1 in ischemic conditions found that HO-1 will significantly reduce infarct volume. Mice that do not have HO-1 will have a larger infarct volume than the wild type [56–58]. Several materials induce HO-1 with promising results in preclinical studies. Some natural ingredients that activate the Nrf-HO-1 pathway, such as dimethyl fumarate, ginkgo biloba, curcumin, polyphenols, and terpenoids, will increase the neuroprotective effect on stroke models [56, 59, 60].

4. Green tea and antioxidant

Green tea is a traditional drink made from the Camellia sinensis tree, which is widely consumed in various countries, especially in Asia. Polyphenols from green tea, especially its active component, namely EGCG (epigallocatechin-3-gallate), have received more attention because they have potential therapeutic agents to prevent neurodegeneration, inflammatory diseases, and cancer [25, 61, 62]. The ability of green tea is mainly due to its antioxidant, free radical scavenger, metal chelation, anticancer, anti-apoptotic, and anti-inflammatory properties [26].

EGCG is roughly composed of four derivatives based on structural variations, including Epicatechin (EC), Epigallocatechin (EGC), Epicatechin gallate (ECG), and epigallocatechin-3-gallate (EGCG). EGCG consists of 10% dry green tea extract and about 50–80% or 200–300 mg of one cup of brewed green tea (**Figure 2**) [26, 63].

The metabolism of green tea polyphenols in the body has been widely studied. It is reported that green tea polyphenols are absorbed, distributed, metabolized, and excreted within 24 hours. In humans, when given 1.2 g of green tea that has been decaffeinated, within 1 hour, it will increase plasma levels by 46–268 ng/ml and excreted in the first 24 hours in the range of 1.6–3.2 mg. Therefore, drinking 6 cups of green tea a day will increase the concentration of green tea polyphenols by 12 times and will be sufficient for antioxidant activity against oxidative damage. These data are then supported by animal studies, where giving green tea 35 mg/kg/day will prevent oxidative damage and memory regression and can delay aging [6, 25, 52, 59, 63].

Free radicals, including ROS and nitrogen species such as NO, superoxide, and hydroxyl free radicals, are naturally produced to support the host defense system against oxidative stress and inflammation stimulated by pathogens and infections. Still, these species have two natural faces, namely, in the event of free radicals that the host produces. Excessive amounts in the body will cause destructive processes that cause DNA, protein, and lipid damage, leading to apoptosis and cell death [65, 66].

DOI: http://dx.doi.org/10.5772/intechopen.107068

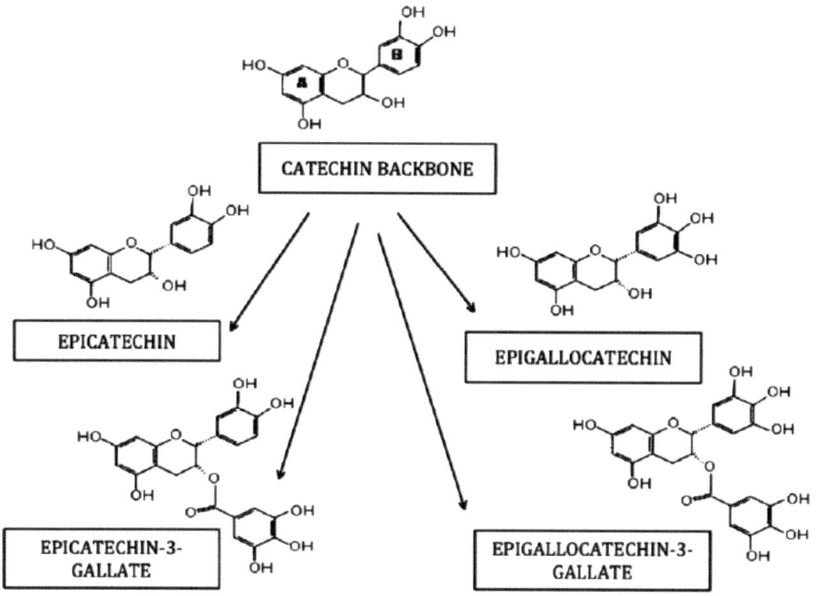

Figure 2.
The structure of green tea catechins and their four derivatives have antioxidant effects, namely Epicatechin, Epigallocatechin, Epicatechin-3-gallate, and epigallocatechin-3-gallate [26, 64].

Green tea polyphenol compounds are biological antioxidants that have a radical scavenger effect. Green tea contains two ingredients that have potent antioxidant properties, namely EGCG and ECG. This antioxidant ability is caused by the presence of ortho-trihydroxy groups in the B chain, 4-keto and 5-hydroxyl in the C chain, and galloyl moiety in the A chain. The difference in antioxidant activity in EGCG and ECG is very slight, which is related to each group's hydroxyl group. Therefore, these molecules can generally clean the radical group 1,1-diphenyl-3-picrylhydrazyl, as well as peroxyl radicals, NO, free fatty radicals, singlet oxygen, peroxynitrite, hydroxyl free radicals, and superoxide anions through three mechanisms, namely, by chelating the metal ion into an inactive form, direct interaction between catechin and peroxyl radicals through electron transfer to prevent DNA damage, and prevent free radical deamination by forming semi-quinone stable radicals [36, 61, 67].

EGCG is reported to be more effective as a radical scavenger when compared to vitamin E and vitamin C. When compared between green tea derivatives, EGCG (epigallocatechin-3-gallate) > ECG (Epicatechin gallate) > EGC (Epigallocatechin) > EC (Epicatechin) has a positive effect. Antioxidant, while EGC > EGCG>EC > EGC has a protective effect in vitro. The ability as a scavenger radical is due to the presence of ortho-3′,4′-dihydroxy moiety groups, or ortho-trihydroxy groups and is not based on steric structure. An increase in the number of hydroxyl groups will increase the strength of EGCG as a radical scavenger because of the presence of three hydroxyl groups in the B chain group and also consisting of galloyl moiety with three hydroxyl groups in the C chain [6, 26, 36, 68].

Oral administration of EGCG in vivo research showed a decrease in lipid peroxide levels by increasing levels of enzymatic and non-enzymatic antioxidants. EGCG can also completely reverse the effect of AlCl3 through its superoxide dismutase activity and by increasing glutathione peroxidase, Cyt-C oxidase, and acetylcholine esterase. The study aimed to see the impact of improving EGCG in rats and found an improvement in the levels of enzymatic and non-enzymatic antioxidants in about 50% of malondialdehyde levels and a 39% decrease in protein carbonyl in both groups of rats. This effect was also obtained by reducing the dose from 100 to 2 mg/KgBW [26].

Consumption of green tea in humans also shows an increase in antioxidant levels in the body. Long-term consumption of green tea as much as 2–3 cups a day is reported to increase antioxidant activity and total polyphenols, accompanied by a decrease in lipid peroxide, glutathione and hydroperoxide levels. This shows that green tea polyphenols such as EGCG can directly or indirectly affect antioxidant levels to reduce oxidative stress [26, 31, 69].

Besides functioning as a radical scavenger, EGCG also has a chelating effect on heavy metals. Two structures give rise to this chelating effect, including ortho-3′,4′-dihydroxy moiety and 4-keto, 3-hydroxyl or 4-keto and 5-hydroxyl moiety groups. This structure serves as a binding point for heavy metal transitions. It neutralizes their activity by converting from the active form to an inactive redox complex and preventing oxidative damage to cells. In vitro studies using astrocyte cultures have demonstrated the ability of many flavonoids to diffuse, which is also supported by in vivo studies. Administration of EGCG orally for 5 to 10 days indicates the presence of these molecules in brain tissue; this shows the ability of EGCG to penetrate the blood–brain barrier [33, 36, 66, 70].

5. Green tea for stroke prevention

As already mentioned, polyphenols from green tea, especially its active component, namely EGCG, have received more attention because of their potential therapeutic agents for preventing neurodegeneration, inflammatory diseases, and cancer [63, 71]. The ability of green tea is mainly due to its antioxidant, free radical scavenger, metal chelation, anti-cancer, anti-apoptotic, and anti-inflammatory properties. In addition, research on EGCG has provided hope about its potential to improve health in old age by enhancing the morphological and functional disorders that occur in normal aging and its ability to suppress cognitive impairment [34].

Polyphenol compounds in green tea are known to have neuroprotective and neurorestorative effects. EGCG has the effect of increasing cell viability, reducing ROS, and increasing levels of stress markers on the endoplasmic reticulum and markers of apoptosis. EGCG also protects against mitochondrial dysfunction, 6-hydroxydopamine (6-OHDA)-induced toxicity, apoptosis induced by oxidative stress in mitochondria, and glutamate excitotoxicity. EGCG also maintains energy in mitochondria and reduces inflammation in brain tissue and damage to neurons. EGCG also has a neurorestorative effect by increasing neurite growth which makes EGCG a potential candidate as a drug that can modify neurological diseases because it has neurorestorative and neuroprotective effects [6, 33, 68].

The active ingredient of green tea, namely EGCG, in addition to reducing and preventing oxidative stress, EGCG can also reduce inflammation. EGCG is a potent leukocyte elastase inhibitor that mediates the activation of MMP-9 and MMP-2, which will trigger inflammation. Oral administration of EGCG will also reduce inflammation in pulmonary fibrosis, block neutrophil-induced angiogenesis, inhibit pro-inflammatory mediators in inflammatory models, and inhibit pro-inflammatory mediators such as dose-dependent myeloperoxidase. This implies that EGCG is an anti-inflammatory agent with therapeutic potential [25, 27, 62].

EGCG was reported to be able to maintain lipid peroxidation and DNA deamination by protecting cells from lipid peroxidation initiators such as t-butylhydroperoxide, 6-hydroxydopamine, iron, ultraviolet radiation, hydrogen peroxide, and 3-hydroxykynurenine. An in vivo study conducted to determine the effect of EGCG on lipid peroxidation showed a significant decrease in lipid peroxidation. This research is done by measuring the levels of Thiobituric reactive substance (TBARS). Simultaneously, with decreased lipid peroxidation levels, several markers of lipid peroxidation, 4-hydroxynonenal and Malonaldehyde, with increased glutathione peroxidase activity and decreased levels of glutathione. This study has implications for the role of EGCG in protecting cells from lipid peroxidation [69, 72–74].

6. Green tea for treatment of acute ischemic stroke

Camellia sinensis with the active ingredient EGCG inhibits neuronal cell death through apoptosis (increased expression of BCL-2 and decreased expression of Caspase-3) and necroptosis (decreased expression of TNFR1 and RIP 3) in the Rattus norvegicus model of Middle Cerebral Artery Occlusion (MCAO) [31].

A study conducted with R. norvegicus model Middle Cerebral Artery Occlusion (MCAO) found the effect of Camelia sinensis with the active ingredient EGCG on HO-1 expression. Inhibition of HO-1 expression started with doses of 1, 20, and 30 mg/kg BW. So that indicates that the antioxidant properties of green tea can inhibit HO-1 expression starting from the lowest dose in this study. The group with 30 mg/KgBW green tea extract intervention also showed a significant difference compared to the control group. Thus, green tea extract and its active ingredient, namely EGCG, showed an inhibitory effect on HO-1 expression. HO-1 protein is an active protein due to oxidative stress through the Nrf-2 pathway; this decrease in HO-1 expression indicates that the administration of green tea extract and its active ingredient (EGCG) can reduce oxidative stress in stroke models [30, 46].

The same study found no difference between the levels of HMGB-1 in control compared to all interventions, and this indicates that neither green tea nor the active ingredient EGCG affects HMGB-1 levels. The results that showed no difference indicated that HMGB1 in this study was secreted passively by stressed cells so that it could not be inhibited by EGCG or green tea extract [30, 46].

C. sinensis with the active ingredient EGCG also influences the expression of TNFR1 in the MCA model. Significant differences in TNFR1 expression in the intervention group of EGCG 20 mg/kgBW, EGCG 30 mg/kgBW, and green tea extract 30 mg/kgBW compared to the control group. The effect of EGCG and green tea extract on decreasing TNFR1 expression started at a dose of EGCG 20 mg/kgBW, and this shows that both green tea extract and its active ingredient, EGCG, can reduce inflammation that occurs in brain tissue affected by stroke. Inflammation is one of the pathways of cell damage caused by ischemia. TNFR1 protein is the primary receptor of TNF- which will cause the active process of necroptosis and inflammation [30].

Furthermore, a decrease in RIP3 expression was found after green tea intervention, either using the active ingredient in the form of EGCG or green tea extract. A significant difference was also found in the RIP3 expression of the intervention group EGCG 20 mg/kgBW, EGCG 30 mg/kgBW, and green tea extract 30 mg/kgBW compared to the control group. RIP3 protein is an executor protein in the apoptotic process, so the decrease in RIP3 expression indicates that EGCG and green tea extract can prevent necroptosis in the MCAO model. The inhibition of RIP3 expression was initiated at a dose of EGCG 20 mg/kgBW. Green tea extract 30 mg/kgBW also has a similar effect to EGCG 30 mg/kgBW [30].

Bcl-2 is a protein that is a major regulator of mitochondrial permeability and the release of pro-apoptotic molecules. BCL-2, together with Bcl-xL, are anti-apoptotic proteins located in mitochondria and endoplasmic reticulum. In mitochondria, BCL-2 maintains mitochondrial integrity and prevents apoptogenic molecules' release [75–78]. *C. sinensis* with the active ingredient EGCG affects the expression of BCL-2. Based on reserch results, there were significant differences in the expression of BCL-2 in all intervention groups compared to the control group. In the intervention group, EGCG 20 mg/kgBW, EGCG 30 mg/kgBW and green tea extract 30 mg/kgBW found a very significant difference when compared to the control. These results indicate that both EGCG and green tea extract can increase anti-apoptotic protein so that it will prevent apoptosis [31].

A significant difference was found in the expression of Caspase-3. Caspase-3 expression was lower in the EGCG 30 mg/kgBW group and the green tea extract group. These results indicate that EGCG and green tea extract can prevent apoptosis by inhibiting the apoptotic execution pathway. The inhibition of this execution pathway is very important because there are three apoptotic pathways: the intrinsic or mitochondrial pathway, the extrinsic pathway, and the granzyme pathway. If one of them is inhibited, other pathways will activate apoptosis, but if the executor caspase is inhibited, the apoptotic pathways that are active can be inhibited. Inhibit the apoptotic pathway by increasing the anti-apoptotic protein or down-regulating the pro-apoptotic protein caspase-3 [30, 63, 66].

Our study also shows that green tea can increase anti-inflammatory mediators that will increase recovery after stroke. We also use animal model and immunohistochemistry to measure CD 206, a marker for M2-type mitochondria. According to our research, there is an increase in CD 206 expression in both Green tea and EGCG group [46, 79].

The study on the benefit of green tea should be conducted in the clinical setting to know about the benefit of green tea in acute ischemic stroke. Its potential benefit can be as an adjunct treatment for acute ischemic stroke besides standard treatment.

7. Summary

The current standard of treatment for acute ischemic stroke is thrombolysis. However, only 2–8.5% of stroke patients can undergo thrombolysis in America, and less than 2% in the world undergo thrombolysis.

Green tea (*C. sinensis*) is the most consumed beverage in the world and is a source of polyphenols known as catechins, including epigallocatechin-3-gallate (EGCG), which is 63% of total catechins.

C. sinensis with the active ingredient EGCG inhibits neuronal cell death through apoptosis (increased expression of BCL-2 and decreased expression of Caspase-3) and necroptosis (decreased expression of TNFR1 and RIP 3) in acute ischemic stroke as in the R. norvegicus model of Middle Cerebral Artery Occlusion (MCAO), it also can decrease necroptossis and increase M2 type microglia.

Author details

Abdulloh Machin[1,2,3] and Shafira Putri Widiawan[1*]

1 Departement Neurology Faculty of Medicine, Universitas Airlangga, Surabaya, Indonesia

2 Dr. Soetomo General Hospital, Surabaya, Indonesia

3 Universitas Airlangga Hospital, Surabaya, Indonesia

*Address all correspondence to: shafira.putri.widiawan-2019@fk.unair.ac.id

References

[1] Caplan LR, Liebeskind DS. 5. Pathology, anatomy, and pathophysiology of stroke. In: Caplan LR, editor. Caplan's Stroke: A Clinical Approach. 5th ed. United Kingdom: Cambridge University Press; 2016. pp. 19-54

[2] Powers WJ, Rabinstein AA, Ackerson T, Adeoye OM, Bambakidis NC, Becker K, et al. Guidelines for the early management of patients with acute ischemic stroke: 2019 update to the 2018 guidelines for the early management of acute ischemic stroke a guideline for healthcare professionals from the American Heart Association/American Stroke A. Stroke. 2019;**50**:344-418

[3] Powers WJ, Rabinstein AA, Ackerson T, Adeoye OM, Bambakidis NC, Becker K, et al. 2018 Guidelines for the early management of patients with acute ischemic stroke: A guideline for healthcare professionals from the american heart Association/ American Stroke Association. Stroke. 2018;**49**:46-110

[4] Feigin VL, Khrisnamurthi RV, Krishnamurthi RV, Khrisnamurthi RV. Global burden of stroke. In: Grotta JC, Albers GW, Broderics JP, editors. Stroke Pathophysiology, Diagnosis, and Management. 6th ed. China: Elsevier Inc.; 2016. pp. 165-206

[5] Ropper AH, Samuel MA, Klein JP. Cerebrovascular disease. In: Adams and Victor's: Principles of Neurology. 10th ed. New York: McGraw Hill; 2014

[6] Pérez A, Santamaria EK, Operario D, Tarkang EE, Zotor FB, Cardoso SR de SN, et al. Stroke Pathophysiology, diagnosi and management. BMC Public Health 2017;5:1-8

[7] Reynolds MA, Kirchick HJ, Dahlen JR, Anderberg JM, McPherson PH, Nakamura KK, et al. Early biomarkers of stroke. Clinical Chemistry. 2003;**49**(10):1733-1739

[8] Scott SE, Zabel K, Collins J, Hobbs KC, Kretschmer MJ, Lach M, et al. First mildly Ill, non-hospitalized case of coronavirus disease 2019 (COVID-19) without viral transmission in the United States - Maricopa county, Arizona, 2020. Clinical Infectious Diseases. 2020;**71**(15):807-812

[9] Howard G, Howard VJ. Stroke Disparities. In: Grotta JC, Albers GW, Broderick JP, Kasner SE, Lo EH, Mendelow AD, et al., editors. Stroke: Pathophysiology, Diagnosis, and Management. 6th ed. China: Elsevier Inc; 2016. pp. 207-216

[10] Coveney S, McCabe JJ, Murphy S, O'Donnell M, Kelly PJ. Anti-inflammatory therapy for preventing stroke and other vascular events after ischaemic stroke or transient ischaemic attack. In: Cochrane Database of Systematic Reviews. Vol. 2020. New Jersey: John Wiley and Sons Ltd; 2020

[11] Deb P, Sharma S, Hassan KM. Pathophysiologic mechanisms of acute ischemic stroke: An overview with emphasis on therapeutic significance beyond thrombolysis. Pathophysiology. 2010;**17**:197-218

[12] Smith MS, Bonomo J, Knight WA, Prestigiacomo CJ, Richards CT, Ramser E, et al. Endovascular therapy for patients with acute ischemic stroke during the COVID-19 pandemic: A proposed algorithm. Stroke 2020;51(6):1902-1909

[13] Lv P, Jin H, Liu Y, Cui W, Peng Q, Liu R, et al. Comparison of risk factor

between lacunar stroke and large artery atherosclerosis stroke: A cross-sectional study in China. PLoS One. 2016;**11**(3):e0149605

[14] Zhang LL, Guo YJ, Lin YP, Hu RZ, Yu JP, Yang J, et al. Stroke care in the first affiliated hospital of Chengdu Medical College during the COVID-19 outbreak. European Neurology. 2020;**83**(6):630-635

[15] Huang WH, Teng LC, Yeh TK, Chen YJ, Lo WJ, Wu MJ, et al. 2019 Novel coronavirus disease (COVID-19) in Taiwan: Reports of two cases from Wuhan, China. Journal of Microbiology, Immunology and Infection. 2020;**53**:481-484

[16] Clark WM, Wechsler LR, Sabounjian LA, Schwiderski UE. Citicoline stroke study G. A phase III randomized efficacy trial of 2000 mg citicoline in acute ischemic stroke patients. Neurology. 2001;**57**(9):1595-1602

[17] Clark WM, Williams BJ, Selzer KA, Zweifler RM, Sabounjian LA, Gammans RE. A randomized efficacy trial of citicoline in patients with acute ischemic stroke. Stroke. 1999;**30**(12):2592-2597

[18] Álvarez-Sabín J, Román GC, Alvarez-Sabin J, Roman GC. The role of citicoline in neuroprotection and neurorepair in ischemic stroke. Brain Sciences. 2013;**3**(3):1395-1414

[19] Secades JJ, Alvarez-Sabin J, Castillo J, Diez-Tejedor E, Martinez-Vila E, Rios J, et al. Citicoline for acute ischemic stroke: A systematic review and formal meta-analysis of randomized, double-blind, and placebo-controlled trials. Journal of Stroke and Cerebrovascular Diseases. 2016;**25**(8):1984-1996

[20] Overgaard K. The effects of citicoline on acute ischemic stroke: A review. Journal of Stroke and Cerebrovascular Diseases. 2014;**23**(7):1764-1769

[21] Elmore S. Apoptosis: A review of programmed cell death. Toxicologic Pathology. 2007;**35**(4):495-516

[22] Ray PD, Huang BW, Tsuji Y. Reactive oxygen species (ROS) homeostasis and redox regulation in cellular signaling. Cellular Signalling. 2012;**24**(5):981-990

[23] Song J, Park J, Oh Y, Lee JE. Glutathione suppresses cerebral infarct volume and cell death after ischemic injury: Involvement of FOXO3 inactivation and Bcl2 expression. Oxidative Medicine and Cellular Longevity. 2015;**2015**:426069

[24] Yu Y, Tang D, Kang R. Oxidative stress-mediated HMGB1 biology. Frontiers in Physiology. 2015;**6**:93

[25] Gundimeda U, McNeill TH, Fan TK, Deng R, Rayudu D, Chen Z, et al. Green tea catechins potentiate the neuritogenic action of brain-derived neurotrophic factor: Role of 67-kDa laminin receptor and hydrogen peroxide. Biochemical and Biophysical Research Communications. 2014;**445**(1):218-224

[26] Kim HS, Quon MJ, Kim JA. New insights into the mechanisms of polyphenols beyond antioxidant properties; lessons from the green tea polyphenol, epigallocatechin 3-gallate. Redox Biology. 2014;**2**:187-195

[27] Rasoolijazi H, Joghataie MT, Roghani M, Nobakht M. The beneficial effect of (−)-epigallocatechin-3-gallate in an experimental model of Alzheimer's disease in rat: A behavioral analysis. Iranian Biomedical Journal. 2007;**11**(4):237-243

[28] Tao L, Park JY, Lambert JD. Differential prooxidative effects

of the green tea polyphenol, (−)-epigallocatechin-3-gallate, in normal and oral cancer cells are related to differences in sirtuin 3 signaling. Molecular Nutrition & Food Research. 2015;**59**(2):203-211

[29] Li MD, Lang M, Deng F, Chang K, Buch K, Rincon S, et al. Analysis of stroke detection during the COVID-19 pandemic using natural language processing of radiology reports. American Journal of Neuroradiology. 2021;**42**(3):429-434

[30] Machin A, Purwanto DA, Nasronuddin, Sugianto P, Aulanni'am A, Subadi I, et al. Camellia sinensis with its active compound egcg can decrease necroptosis via inhibition of ho-1 expression. EurAsian Journal of Biosciences. 2020;**14**(1):1813-1820

[31] Machin A, Susilo I, Purwanto DA. Green tea and its active compound epigallocathechin-3-gallate (EGCG) inhibit neuronal apoptosis in a middle cerebral artery occlusion (MCAO) model. Journal of Basic and Clinical Physiology and Pharmacology. 2021;**32**(4):319-325

[32] Kim Y, Lee J. Effect of (−)-epigallocatechin-3-gallate on anti-inflammatory response via heme oxygenase-1 induction during adipocyte-macrophage interactions. Food Science and Biotechnology. 2016;**25**(6):1767-1773

[33] Yao K, Ye P, Zhang L, Tan J, Tang X, Zhang Y. Epigallocatechin gallate protects against oxidative stress-induced mitochondria-dependent apoptosis in human lens epithelial cells. Molecular Vision. 2008;**14**:217-223

[34] Kim E, Han SY, Hwang K, Kim D, Kim EM, Hossain MA, et al. Antioxidant and cytoprotective effects of (-)-Epigallocatechin-3-(3"-O-methyl) gallate. International Journal of Molecular Sciences. 2019;**20**(16):2-13

[35] Gao Z, Han Y, Hu Y, Wu X, Wang Y, Zhang X, et al. Targeting HO-1 by Epigallocatechin-3-gallate reduces contrast-induced renal injury via anti-oxidative stress and anti-inflammation pathways. PLoS One. 2016;**11**(2):1-17

[36] Li W, Zhu S, Li J, Assa A, Jundoria A, Xu J, et al. EGCG stimulates autophagy and reduces cytoplasmic HMGB1 levels in endotoxin-stimulated macrophages. Biochemical Pharmacology. 2011;**81**(9):1152-1163

[37] Mahler A, Mandel S, Lorenz M, Ruegg U, Wanker EE, Boschmann M, et al. Epigallocatechin-3-gallate: A useful, effective and safe clinical approach for targeted prevention and individualised treatment of neurological diseases? The EPMA Journal. 2013;**4**(1):5

[38] Guo Y, Li P, Guo Q, Shang K, Yan D, Du S, et al. Pathophysiology and biomarkers in acute ischemic stroke – A review. Tropical Journal of Pharmaceutical Research. 2013;**12**(6):1097-1105

[39] Zhang H, Ofengeim D, Shi Y, Zhang F, Hwang JY, Chen J, et al. Molecular and cellular mechanisms of ischemia-induced neuronal death. In: Grotta JC, Albers GW, Broderick JP, Kasner SE, Lo EH, Mendelow AD, et al., editors. Stroke: Pathophysiology, Diagnosis, and Management. 6th ed. China: Elsevier Inc; 2016. pp. 60-79

[40] Zhai D-X, Kong Q-F, Xu W-S, Bai S-S, Peng H-S, Zhao K, et al. RAGE expression is up-regulated in human cerebral ischemia and pMCAO rats. Neuroscience Letters. 2008;**445**(1):117-121

[41] Murray KN, Parry-Jones AR, Allan SM. Interleukin-1 and acute

brain injury. Frontiers in Cellular Neuroscience. 2015;**9**:18

[42] Ahmad I, Rathore FA. Neurological manifestations and complications of COVID-19: A literature review. Journal of Clinical Neuroscience. 2020;**77**:8-12

[43] Vanlangenakker N, Vanden Berghe T, Krysko DV, Festjens N, Vandenabeele P. Molecular mechanisms and pathophysiology of necrotic cell death. Current Molecular Medicine. 2008;**8**(3):207-220

[44] Nikoletopoulou V, Markaki M, Palikaras K, Tavernarakis N. Crosstalk between apoptosis, necrosis and autophagy. Biochimica et Biophysica Acta. 2013;**1833**(12):3448-3459

[45] Chen PM, Hemmen TM. Evolving healthcare delivery in neurology during the coronavirus disease 2019 (COVID-19) pandemic. Frontiers in Neurology. 2020;**11**:578

[46] MacHin A, Divamillenia D, Fatimah N, Susilo I, Purwanto D, Subadi I, et al. The effect of green tea with EGCG active compound in enhancing the expression of M2 microglia marker (CD206). Neurology India. 2022;**70**(2):530-534

[47] Levine SR. Pathophysiology and therapeutic targets for ischemic stroke. Clinical Cardiology. 2004;**27**(5 Suppl. 2): 12-24

[48] Ayala A, Munoz MF, Arguelles S. Lipid peroxidation: Production, metabolism, and signaling mechanisms of malondialdehyde and 4-hydroxy-2-nonenal. Oxidative Medicine and Cellular Longevity. 2014;**2014**:360438

[49] Touyz RM, Briones AM. Reactive oxygen species and vascular biology: Implications in human hypertension. Hypertension Research. 2011;**34**(1):5-14

[50] Lewén A, Fujimura M, Sugawara T, Matz P, Copin J, Chan PH. Oxidative stress – dependent release of mitochondrial cytochrome c after traumatic brain injury. 2001:914-920

[51] Setyowatie S, MacHin A, Aulia NN. Association between bleeding volume with heme oxygenase-1 and malondialdehyde levels in patients of acute intracerebral hemorrhage. Gaceta médica de Caracas. 2021;**129**(Supl 2):S373-S378

[52] He F, Zhang Y, Chen S, Ye B, Chen J, Li C. Effect of EGCG on oxidative stress and Nrf2/HO-1 pathway in neurons exposed to oxygen-glucose deprivation/reperfusion. Zhong Nan Da Xue Xue Bao. Yi Xue Ban. 2018;**43**(10):1041-1047

[53] Liu C, Zhu C, Wang G, Xu R, Zhu Y. Higenamine regulates Nrf2-HO-1-Hmgb1 axis and attenuates intestinal ischemia-reperfusion injury in mice. Inflammation Research. 2015;**64**(6):395-403

[54] Saleem S, Zhuang H, Biswal S, Christen Y, Dore S. On heme oxygenase 1 in ischemic reperfusion. Brain Injury. 2008:3389-3396

[55] Iii RHL, Chen R, Selim MH, Hanafy KA. Heme oxygenase-1-mediated neuroprotection in subarachnoid hemorrhage via intracerebroventricular deferoxamine. Journal of Neuroinflammation. 2016;**13**(1):1-15

[56] Bereczki D Jr, Balla J, Bereczki D. Heme oxygenase-1: Clinical relevance in ischemic stroke. Current Pharmaceutical Design. 2018;**24**(20):2229-2235

[57] Kim SJ, Eum HA, Billiar TR, Lee SM. Role of heme oxygenase 1 in TNF/TNF receptor-mediated apoptosis after hepatic ischemia/reperfusion in rats. Shock. 2013;**39**(4):380-388

[58] Kishimoto Y, Kondo K, Momiyama Y. The protective role of heme oxygenase-1 in atherosclerotic diseases. International Journal of Molecular Sciences. 2019;**20**(15):1-15

[59] Afonso MB, Rodrigues PM, Simao AL, Ofengeim D, Carvalho T, Amaral JD, et al. Activation of necroptosis in human and experimental cholestasis. Cell Death & Disease. 2016;**7**(9):e2390

[60] LeBlanc RH 3rd, Chen R, Selim MH, Hanafy KA. Heme oxygenase-1-mediated neuroprotection in subarachnoid hemorrhage via intracerebroventricular deferoxamine. Journal of Neuroinflammation. 2016;**13**(1):244

[61] Ran ZH, Xu Q, Tong JL, Xiao SD. Apoptotic effect of Epigallocatechin-3-gallate on the human gastric cancer cell line MKN45 via activation of the mitochondrial pathway. World Journal of Gastroenterology. 2007;**13**(31):4255-4259

[62] Kim E, Han SY, Hwang K, Kim D, Kim E, Hossain MA, et al. Antioxidant and cytoprotective effects of (−)-Epigallocatechin-3- (3″ - O -methyl) gallate. 2019;**20**(16):1-13

[63] Yao C, Zhang J, Liu G, Chen F, Lin Y. Neuroprotection by (−)-epigallocatechin-3-gallate in a rat model of stroke is mediated through inhibition of endoplasmic reticulum stress. Molecular Medicine Reports. 2014;**9**(1):69-76

[64] Lim SH, Kim HS, Kim YK, Kim TM, Im S, Chung ME, et al. The functional effect of epigallocatechin gallate on ischemic stroke in rats. Acta Neurobiologiae Experimentalis (Wars). 2010;**70**(1):40-46

[65] Gao Z, Han Y, Hu Y, Wu X, Wang Y, Zhang X, et al. Targeting HO-1 by Epigallocatechin-3-gallate reduces contrast-induced renal injury via anti-oxidative stress and anti-inflammation pathways. PLoS One. 2016;**11**(2):e0149032

[66] Ye P, Lin K, Li Z, Liu J, Yao K, Xu W. (−)-Epigallocatechin gallate regulates expression of apoptotic genes and protects cultured human lens epithelial cells under hyperglycemia. Molecular Biology. 2013;**47**(2):251-257

[67] Zhu W, Xu J, Ge Y, Cao H, Ge X, Luo J, et al. Epigallocatechin-3-gallate (EGCG) protects skin cells from ionizing radiation via heme oxygenase-1 (HO-1) overexpression. Journal of Radiation Research. 2014;**55**(6):1056-1065

[68] Ekker MS, Boot EM, Singhal AB, Tan KS, Debette S, Tuladhar AM, et al. Epidemiology, aetiology, and management of ischaemic stroke in young adults. Lancet Neurology. 2018;**17**(9):790-801

[69] Wang ZM, Gao W, Wang H, Zhao D, Nie ZL, Shi JQ, et al. Green tea polyphenol epigallocatechin-3-gallate inhibits TNF-alpha-induced production of monocyte chemoattractant protein-1 in human umbilical vein endothelial cells. Cellular Physiology and Biochemistry. 2014;**33**(5):1349-1358

[70] Snitsarev V, Young MN, Miller RM, Rotella DP. The spectral properties of (−)-epigallocatechin 3-O-gallate (EGCG) fluorescence in different solvents: dependence on solvent polarity. PLoS One. 2013;**8**(11):e79834

[71] Singh BN, Shankar S, Srivastava RK. Green tea catechin, epigallocatechin-3-gallate (EGCG): mechanisms, perspectives and clinical applications. Biochemical Pharmacology. 2011;**82**(12):1807-1821

[72] Jiang J, Mo ZC, Yin K, Zhao GJ, Lv YC, Ouyang XP, et al. Epigallocatechin-3-gallate prevents TNF-α-induced NF-κB activation thereby upregulating ABCA1 via the Nrf2/Keap1 pathway in macrophage foam cells. International Journal of Molecular Medicine. 2012;**29**(5):946-956

[73] Leu JG, Lin CY, Jian JH, Shih CY, Liang YJ. Epigallocatechin-3-gallate combined with alpha lipoic acid attenuates high glucose-induced receptor for advanced glycation end products (RAGE) expression in human embryonic kidney cells. Anais da Academia Brasileira de Ciências. 2013;**85**(2):745-752

[74] Yang WS, Moon SY, Lee MJ, Park SK. Epigallocatechin-3-gallate attenuates the effects of TNF-α in vascular endothelial cells by causing ectodomain shedding of TNF receptor 1. Cellular Physiology and Biochemistry. 2016;**38**(5):1963-1974

[75] Cai J, Yang J, Jones DP. Mitochondrial control of apoptosis: The role of cytochrome c. Biochim Biophys Acta - Bioenergetics. 1998;**1366**(1-2):139-149

[76] Gogvadze V, Orrenius S, Zhivotovsky B. Multiple pathways of cytochrome c release from mitochondria in apoptosis. Biochim Biophys Acta - Bioenergetics. 2006;**1757**(5-6):639-647

[77] Sinkovics JG. Programmed cell death (apoptosis): its virological and immunological connections (a review). Acta Microbiologica Hungarica. 1991;**38**(3-4):321-334

[78] Wang C, Youle RJ. The role of mitochondria in apoptosis*. Annual Review of Genetics. 2009;**43**:95-118

[79] Machin A, Syaharani R, Susilo I, Hamdan M, Fauziah D, Purwanto DA. The effect of Camellia sinensis (green tea) with its active compound EGCG on neuronal cell necroptosis in Rattus norvegicus middle cerebral artery occlusion (MCAO) model. Journal of Basic and Clinical Physiology and Pharmacology. 2021;**32**(4):527-531

Chapter 5

Research Progress on the Health Benefits of Scented Tea

Bowen Liu, Jun Zhang, Xiaojian Zhou, Shuduan Deng and Guanben Du

Abstract

Scented tea, also known as fragrant tea, mainly comprises green tea as the tea base and the dried and processed flowers of various plants. It is a unique reprocessed tea in China. There are many types of scented tea, including jasmine, lily, osmanthus, rose and honeysuckle. The scenting process greatly influences the quality of the scented tea. Humidifying continuous scenting processes, frying flower processes and innovative drying methods have been developed to resolve the issues of cumbersome, time-consuming and low utilisation rates of flowers in the process of making scented tea. The main chemical components of scented tea are polyphenols as well as exogenous plant glycosides, flavonoids, lactones, coumarins, quercetin, steroids, terpenoids and other compounds. Scented tea plays an active role in the prevention and treatment of various diseases and has as anti-oxidant, anti-cancer, hypoglycaemic, hypolipidemic, immunomodulatory and neuromodulatory effects. This chapter mainly reviews and summarises the types of scented teas and their related health functions.

Keywords: scented tea, medicinal value, tea polyphenols, health function, disease prevention

1. Introduction

Scented tea, also known as fragrant tea, is made from the flowers or leaves of plants. It is a type of reprocessed tea unique to China. It uses the properties of tea that make it good at absorbing odours and blends scented flowers and tea together. The tea absorbs the fragrance and then the dried flowers are removed using a sieve. The resulting scented tea has a strong fragrance and a bright tea drink. Scented tea has a long history of production. As early as the Song Dynasty, spices were added to green tea as a tribute to the emperor [1]. The processing technology of tea gradually matured during the Ming Dynasty and the scenting method of scented tea has since progressed [2]. The quality of scented tea is related to the scenting process. Mature scenting processes, such as moisturising continuous scenting, frying flower processes and innovative drying methods can be used to ensure that the scented tea maintains appropriate water content during the scenting process and improves the ability of the tea base to absorb the fragrance of the flowers. Chinese scented tea is mainly produced in the Guangxi, Fujian, Yunnan, Sichuan and Chongqing provinces. In 2021, the scented tea output in China was 2.917 million tonnes. Scented tea has been exported to Japan, the USA, Russia, Germany and other countries for many years and has a good reputation in local markets.

Scented tea contains various nutrients, such as proteins, amino acids, tea polyphenols, tea polysaccharides, vitamins and minerals. It also contains pigments, taste substances amino acids, catechins, caffeine and aroma substances. These substances not only improve the quality of scented tea but are also required for human physiological activities and contribute to the health effects of scented tea. Protein and amino acids are essential components of human metabolism. The water-soluble protein content of scented tea is around 2% and can be directly absorbed and used by the body through drinking the tea [3]. Scented tea is rich in amino acids, including theanine, glutamic acid and aspartic acid as well as vitamins. For example, jasmine scented tea contains 80–90 mg of vitamin C per 100 g of jasmine scented tea and can improve the immune system [4]. Scented tea also contains mineral elements, such as phosphorus, potassium, calcium, sodium, magnesium and sulphur as well as trace elements, such as iron, manganese, zinc, selenium, fluorine and iodine. In addition, the polyphenolic compounds, tea polysaccharides, caffeine and other components present in scented tea have good health effects on human physiological activities [5]. Scented tea also contains aromatic substances, including esters, alcohols and hydrocarbons, among which linalool, indole, benzyl alcohol and methyl salicylate are the main aroma components. These aromatic substances can aid digestion, relieve stomach pain and calm and regulate the nervous system [6]. Scented tea has the same refreshing effects as coffee due to its high content of caffeine and alkaloids, which are central nervous system stimulants. However, drinking coffee regularly may cause arteriosclerosis, whereas drinking scented tea can avoid this adverse effect. Scented tea contains polyphenols and vitamin C, which can effectively eliminate the adverse effects of caffeine. On the other hand, the caffeine in scented tea can promote gastric secretion, help digestion, enhance fat metabolism and effectively reduce body mass index [7]. Therefore, scented tea can also be used to promote weight loss. Scented tea contains a large amount of vitamin A, vitamin C and other trace elements that protect the eyes and have therapeutic effects on dry eyes caused by overuse of the eyes. Traditional Chinese medicine also commonly uses scented tea for the treatment of eye diseases [8]. Several cell and animal studies have shown that tea polyphenols, polysaccharides and pigments have significant anti-cancer and anti-tumour effects. The main anti-cancer pathways include inhibiting cancer cell proliferation, regulation of signalling pathways to induce apoptosis of cancer cells, inhibition of angiogenesis, inhibition of metastasis and infection of cancer cells and inhibition of tumour immune escape mechanism [9–11].

The pharmacologist Li Shizhen's 'Compendium of Materia Medica' also records the health care effects of scented tea. The chemical composition and health functions of scented tea have been extensively studied over the past two decades to examine the mechanisms behind the health benefits of scented tea. The scientific community and mass media have gradually begun to pay attention to the beneficial properties of scented tea. For example, drinking scented tea is associated with anti-oxidant [12], anti-cancer [13], hypoglycaemic [14], hypolipidaemic [15], immunomodulatory [16] and neuromodulatory [17] effects. This chapter mainly reviews and discusses the health functions related to scented tea and the direction of future research and development.

2. Types of scented tea

Types of scented tea mainly include jasmine, lily, osmanthus, rose and honeysuckle, as shown in **Figure 1**.

2.1 Jasmine scented tea

Jasmine scented tea is mainly produced in the Guangxi, Fujian, Sichuan and Yunnan provinces of China. It is a reprocessed tea made by blending tea with jasmine flowers. When brewed and consumed, its aroma is strong, fresh and refreshing. Jasmine scented tea generally uses green tea as the tea base. The choice of tea base is an important factor in determining the quality of jasmine scented tea. The aroma and taste of jasmine scented tea can be improved by making jasmine scented tea with green tea scraps of different particle sizes [18]. Different drying methods lead to changes in the surface and microstructure of the tea base, which in turn affect the quality of the finished jasmine tea. The emergence of vacuum freeze-drying technology has resolved this issue and the moisture content and overall quality of tea base have reached controllable conditions. Therefore, the quality of jasmine tea after scenting is better than that prepared by hot air drying [19].

Jasmine scented tea has physiological effects as well as significant health care properties. Studies have shown that jasmine scented tea can help obese people to reduce lipid levels and lose weight [20, 21]. Improved living conditions have led to women focusing more on ageing and skin problems. The anti-ageing and anti-oxidant health effects of jasmine tea also play an important role in the health benefits of jasmine tea. The polyphenols and pigments in jasmine tea have anti-bacterial effects. Gargling with the water extract of jasmine scented tea can resolve oral problems, such as oral ulcers and swollen gums.

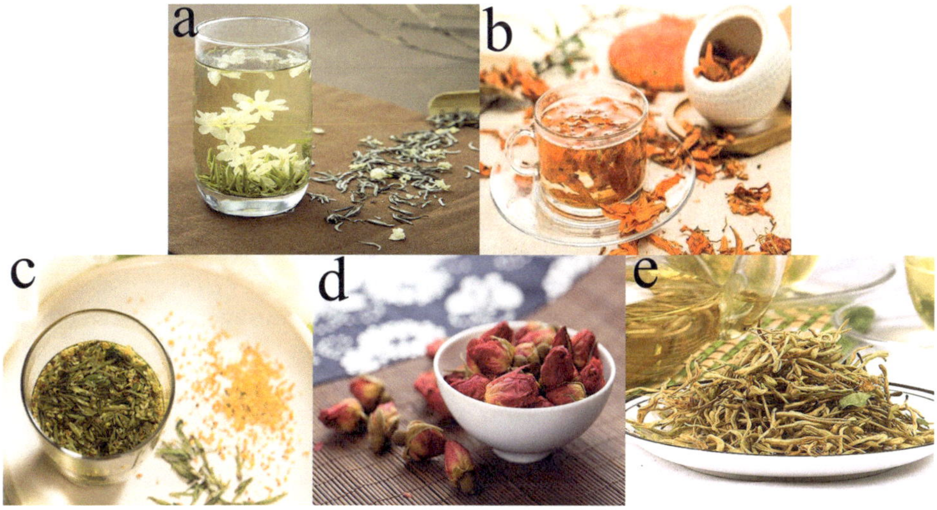

Figure 1.
Different types of scented tea. (a) Jasmine, (b) lily, (c) osmanthus, (d) rose, and (e) honeysuckle scented teas.

2.2 Lily scented tea

Lily scented tea is mainly produced in the Anhui, Jiangsu and Guangdong provinces. Lily scented tea is prepared by processing fresh lily and green tea together, which retains the original biological activity factor of lily and has the fragrance of green tea. In addition to its strong aroma, lily has edible and medicinal properties. After scenting is complete, the flowers are mixed with tea, dried and packaged together, which improves the quality of scented tea and enhances its edible and medicinal value. Current methods of lily scented tea preparation include the treatment of tea billet, maintenance of flowers and the triple scenting of flowers. Finally, high-quality lily and dried tea greens are mixed for drying. This method can control the water content of lily scented tea, improve the quality and taste of lily scented tea and improve its medicinal value [22]. During the traditional drying process of flowers and tea, secondary drying reduces the fragrance of flowers and affects the quality of scented tea, while processing technologies, such as microwave drying or the use of desiccants, can greatly reduce the loss of floral fragrance [23].

Lily scented tea has high nutritional and medicinal values. While it is often made into desserts, people in the Guangdong region prefer to use it to make a tea drink to relieve coughing and sputum production. Lily scented tea tastes sweet and has no irritating taste. It moistens the lungs to stop coughing, clears away heart-burn and calms the mind. Lily scented tea is nourishing and medicinal and can be consumed all year round. It contains a variety of alkaloids, which have a preventive effect on leukopenia, increases the red blood cell count in the blood and has therapeutic effects on cytopenia after chemotherapy and radiotherapy [24, 25]. Lily scented tea can also improve the immune system and has preventive effects on a variety of cancers. The 'Compendium of Materia Medica' states that lily scented tea is a high-quality tonic and has properties similar to those of ginseng in tea.

2.3 Rose scented tea

Rose scented tea is mainly produced in the Guangdong and Fujian provinces in China. It is one of women's favourite scented teas and is also the most common scented tea. Brewed rose scented tea exudes a refreshing aroma and refreshes the consumer. The quality of the finished product of rose scented tea is related to the processing technology. The type of rose and tea base used during the process directly affects the quality of scented tea. During the scenting process, freeze-dried roses are selected and mixed with green tea for secondary scenting. Airtight conditions are maintained during the scenting process to ensure an appealing drinking taste and aroma. Nutrients are not lost during scenting, improving the medicinal value [26]. The tea needs to be dried after scenting. Microwave technology can preserve the fragrance of the scented tea to a great extent and resolve issues such as dull colour and loss of aroma of the scented tea due to high temperature and humidity during drying using the traditional process [27].

Rose scented tea is a precious medicinal material and traditional Chinese medicine often uses rose scented tea with other traditional Chinese medicines to produce different formulas. Using rose scented tea to make wine can reduce blood lipid levels, improve vitality and improve skin texture [28]. Rose essential oil refined from rose scented tea can promote the development of male hormones and sperm and promote blood circulation and metabolism. Rose scented tea is also a commonly used a gynaecological Chinese medicine and has a significant effects in the treatment of gynaecological diseases [29]. Recent studies have shown that rose scented tea extract has anti-viral effects and has been used in the treatment of acquired immune deficiency syndrome and leukaemia and has achieved remarkable results.

2.4 Honeysuckle scented tea

Honeysuckle is a type of vine that is widely used in the pharmaceutical, food and chemical industries [30–32]. Honeysuckle scented tea is prepared by combining fried green tea and fresh honeysuckle in a sealer, separating the green tea and honeysuckle with gauze and stacking them in multiple layers to fully mix the honeysuckle and tea. Finally, dried honeysuckle and green tea are mixed and packaged. This process gives the tea a strong aroma and medicinal properties.

Honeysuckle is commonly used as a precious Chinese medicine. It is used to reduce fever and toxins, free the channels and improve circulation and has broad-spectrum anti-bacterial and anti-viral effects. More than 70% of cold medicines and anti-inflammatory patented Chinese medicines contain honeysuckle, which is known as 'Chinese medicine antibiotics' and 'green antibiotics'. In addition to its medicinal properties, honeysuckle scented tea is used for beauty, weight loss and health care and has also been shown to protect and repair the body. Honeysuckle scented tea relieves heat stroke, sobers up individuals after consuming alcohol, clears the mind, relieves thirst, removes toxic substances from the body, lowers fat levels, reduces body weight, clears the skin, prevents ageing and increases longevity [33–35]. It can also lower blood pressure, lower serum cholesterol, increase coronary blood flow, prevent coronary heart disease and heart pain and inhibit the formation of cerebral thrombosis. Drinking honeysuckle scented tea can also improve the body's resistance to hypoxic free radicals, delay ageing, improve microcirculation, remove peroxidised fat deposits and promote metabolism.

3. Chemical constituents of scented tea

Polyphenols are an important component of tea, accounting for around 18–36% of the tea dry weight. Catechins are the main components of tea polyphenols, accounting for around 70–80% of the total tea polyphenols. Catechins can be categorised according to molecular structure into four types: epicatechin, epigallocatechin, epicatechin-3-gallate and epigallocatechin-3-gallate as shown in **Figure 2**. Tea polyphenols have strong anti-oxidant effects that are significantly greater than those of vitamins C and E, although they have synergistic effects with vitamin C and E, with anti-ageing effects [36, 37].

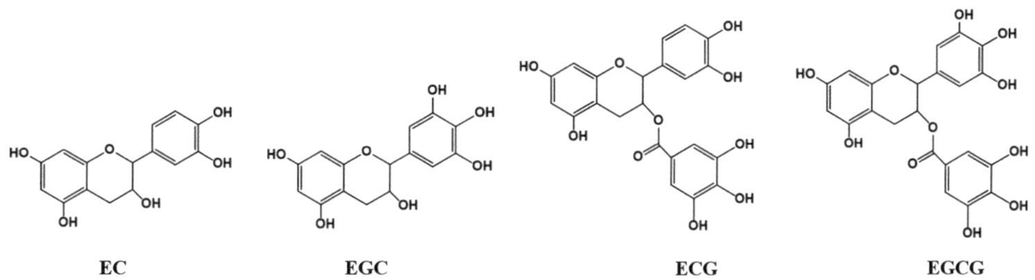

Figure 2.
Structure of catechins EC, epicatechin; EGC, epigallocatechin; ECG, epicatechin-3-gallate and EGCG, epigallocatechin-3-gallate.

In addition to polyphenols, the chemical constituents of scented tea also include glycosides, flavonoids, lactones, coumarins, quercetin, terpenes and other compounds. Chemical studies on jasmine have shown that the main functional components of jasmine include nearly 100 compounds, such as volatile oils, fatty acids, glycosides, terpenoids, lignans and alkaloids [38]. According to the 'Compendium of Materia Medica', decoction of jasmine can be used to treat dysentery and abdominal pain and can also be used as an eye wash to treat conjunctivitis [39].

The chemical constituents of lily scented tea were examined by ethanol reflux extraction and the main components were found to be β-sitosterol, stigmasterol and emodin [40]. Among these, β-sitosterol lowers cholesterol, relieves cough and eliminates phlegm, inhibits tumour formation and inhibits skin ulceration. Sterols have high nutritional value and strong physiological activity and are commonly used in the pharmaceutical, cosmetics, animal growth regulators and food industries. Emodin can be used as a laxative and has anti-bacterial, anti-cough, anti-tumour and blood pressure lowering effects.

Studies on the chemical constituents of osmanthus scented tea show that the volatile components mainly include hexadecanoic acid, methyl docosatrienoate, camphor oil and isomenthone [41]. Studies have shown that the flavonoids in osmanthus scented tea have good anti-bacterial activity, especially against *Escherichia coli* and *Staphylococcus aureus*. Studies on melanin derived from osmanthus scented tea seed coat showed that it has good anti-oxidant activity and can effectively prevent skin ageing [42].

Rose scented tea is rich in vitamins A, B and C and as well as amino acids, polysaccharides, alkaloids and other functional ingredients. The vitamin C content of roses is very high and can reach eight times that of kiwifruit, 20 times that of sea buckthorn and 700 times that of apples. Rose scented tea contains 16.33% protein and is rich in amino acids. Rose also contains a variety of unsaturated acids, including the essential fatty acids linoleic acid, linolenic acid and oleic acid, which together account for 99.75% of the total unsaturated fatty acids [43]. Rose is rich in dietary fibre, rose flavonoids and amino acids and can reduce blood lipids and blood sugar. It is also rich in trace elements including zinc, copper and manganese. These are important elements of superoxide dismutase and selenium, which is an important element of thiooxyreductase and glutathione peroxidase. These enzymes can improve the immune system and have good anti-oxidant effects [44].

The active components of honeysuckle mainly include phenolic acids, flavonoids, volatile oils and triterpenoid saponins, among which phenolic acids are important secondary metabolites in honeysuckle [45, 46]. Honeysuckle has good anti-oxidant activity due to its multiple phenolic hydroxyl groups in the structure [47]. Honeysuckle scented tea contains quercetin, luteolin, kaempferol, β-sitosterol, wogonin and other components, giving it fever-reducing and cleansing properties. It has also been shown to have preventive effects on coronavirus disease 2019 [48].

4. Health functions of scented tea

4.1 Anti-oxidant effects

The anti-oxidant effects of scented tea can be attributed to the polyphenols in the tea and vitamins, flavonoids and phenols in the different scents. Ma et al. [12] found that jasmine scented tea contained large amounts of tea polyphenols compared with black and green teas and its anti-oxidant effects were greater that of vitamin C, as determined using the diphenyl-picrohydrazide method. Cong et al. [49] supplemented the diets of growing rats with 6% jasmine scented tea for 30 days and reported an significantly increased activity of anti-oxidant enzymes in the serum and liver. In addition, jasmine scented tea extract has significant anti-oxidant and anti-ageing effects on ageing mice [50]. A study on the anti-oxidant effect of healthy rabbits in vitro showed that the polar components of osmanthus tea can effectively remove superoxide ions in the body and lipid peroxidation of mitochondria in vitro [51]. Chen et al. [52] reported that 6 weeks of continuous gavage using rose scented tea in restraint stressed mice significantly increased the reduced liver catalase activity and glutathione content observed due to restraint stress and decreased plasma homocysteine levels by 20%. In addition, roses contain a large amount of vitamin C, which is a water-soluble vitamin with strong anti-oxidant activity that can effectively eliminate free radicals. After binding with free radicals, vitamin C can be transformed into dehydroascorbic acid and monohydroascorbic acid to eliminate free radicals, giving roses their anti-oxidant effect [43].

4.2 Anti-cancer effects

Scented tea has inhibitory effects on various cancers, such as liver, skin, stomach, lung, oral, breast, pancreatic and colon cancers [53–55], due to the presence of polyphenols and their oxidation products and caffeine. Tea polyphenols have strong anti-oxidant properties, scavenge free radicals in the body and can block the synthesis of carcinogens, such as ammonium nitrite. The inhibitory effects of scented tea on cancer are achieved via anti-oxidation, induction of apoptosis and regulation of gene expression. In addition, scented tea contains a large amount of chlorogenic acid and related derivatives, which have shown anti-cancer activity against U937 human histiocytic lymphoma cells, KB human oral cancer cells, MCF-7 breast cancer cells and WI38 lung fibroblast cells [56]. Chlorogenic acid can inhibit colon cancer by inducing the production of reactive oxygen species, lung cancer cells by affecting the expression of apoptosis-related genes and liver, oral, gastric, cervical and breast cancers [57–59]. Kawabata et al. [60] used azomethane to induce a rat model of colon cancer and found that ferulic acid could reduce the incidence of colon cancer in rats. Protocatechuic acid can reduce the enzyme activity of MCF-7, A549 non-small cell lung cancer cells, HepG2 human liver cancer cells, HeLa cervical cancer cells and LNCaP prostate cancer cells, effectively penetrate cancer cells, inhibit lactate dehydrogenase activity and damage the mitochondrial membrane potential and also inhibit MMP-2 secretion to prevent its metastasis in human gastric cancer AGS cells [61]. Studies have found that caffeic acid mainly exerts its anti-cancer effects by affecting the mRNA regulatory network and up-regulating levels of mitochondrial reactive oxygen species in tumour cells [62]. Studies have also shown that isochlorogenic acid A has an inhibitory effect on human ovarian cancer cells, skin melanoma cells, central nervous system tumour cells and colorectal cancer cells [63].

4.3 Hypoglycaemic effects

Diabetes is one of the most common chronic diseases seen in clinical medicine its the incidence has gradually increased in young people. The blood glucose levels of individuals fluctuate; however, stable blood glucose levels are an important evaluation index of individual physical health. Scented tea can improve the ability of vanadate to regulate blood glucose. Vanadate suspended in jasmine scented tea has hypoglycaemic effects and can stably and effectively maintain blood glucose at a normal levels within a few weeks [64]. Studies have shown that drinking jasmine scented tea significantly reduces blood glucose [18]. Starch (polysaccharide) in food is digested into oligosaccharides by salivary amylase and pancreatic amylase, converted to glucose by α-glucosidase in the small intestine and finally absorbed. Studies have found that osmanthus tea extract has an inhibitory effect on α-glucosidase [65]. The presence of phenolic compounds in honeysuckle scented tea extract was shown to reduce blood sugar levels in sucrose hyperglycaemic mice and an alloxan diabetes mouse model [66].

4.4 Lipid-lowering effects

Caffeine in tea can reduce the concentration of triglycerides in blood and catechin can inhibit lipid synthesis. The comprehensive effects of caffeine, catechin, tea polysaccharide, cholestenone, inositol, folic acid and pantothenic acid in tea can prevent and inhibit obesity. Studies have shown that the effect of jasmine scented tea on weight control may be related to its ability to increase lipoxin levels [64]. Consumption of jasmine scented tea can prevent elevated blood lipid levels and atherosclerosis, reduce the content of molecular substances in plasma and protect organs, such as the liver and kidneys. A study on rose scented tea found that its lipid-lowering effect mainly comes from its high content of dietary fibre, rose flavonoids and various amino acids [67]. Rose scented tea is rich in dietary fibre, which cannot be converted to glucose in the human body, and has a low glycaemic index. It may be used as a common food for patients with diabetes. Dietary fibre can also combine with bile salts (metabolites of cholesterol), which are then excreted, effectively reducing the concentration of cholesterol in serum and further preventing and treating cardiovascular and cerebrovascular diseases. In addition, dietary fibre also promotes gastrointestinal motility, which can effectively prevent constipation and reduce the incidence of intestinal cancer. Lan et al. [68] examined the effects of rose extract on blood sugar and glucose tolerance in diabetic mice and found that both rose liquid extract and alcohol extract could effectively reduce blood sugar and improve glucose tolerance. A dose effect was seen and rose alcohol extract exerted a greater lipid-lowering effect than rose water extract. A previous study evaluated the lipid-lowering effects of water-extracted flavonoids from honeysuckle and found that they significantly reduced plasma triglyceride and plasma cholesterol levels in hyperglycaemic mice [69]. The mechanisms involved changes in the transcription and expression levels of insulin receptor substrate 1, low density lipoprotein receptor, apolipoprotein 1, fatty acid synthase and cholesterol regulatory element binding protein 2 in the liver of the mouse model. These studies indicate that the polysaccharides, amino acids and flavonoids contained in jasmine, rose and honeysuckle have lipid-lowering effects and that these active substances are likely to have synergistic effects with the polyphenols in green tea in reducing blood lipids.

4.5 Immunoregulation effects

The immune system provides resistance to disease. Researchers at the Fujian Institute of Traditional Chinese Medicine studied the immune function of scented tea on animals. Jasmine scented tea was shown to increase the number of white blood cells, lymphocytes and T lymphocytes in the blood [16]. Lin et al. [70] compared the effects of jasmine scented tea, traditional Chinese medicine (the main components are angelica, yam and liquorice) and compound tea (88.5% scented tea and 11.5% of traditional Chinese medicine) on the immune function of mice with acute renal failure. The results showed that 2.5% scented tea, 2.5% compound tea and 0.3% traditional Chinese medicine could significantly reduce the content of molecular substances in serum and significantly promote the proliferation of mouse spleen T and B lymphocytes and enhance the activity of mouse spleen lymphocytes. The study further showed that jasmine scented tea, traditional Chinese medicine and compound tea could enhance the immune function of the spleen in mice and jasmine scented tea and compound tea had more significant immune effects on mice. In addition, Li et al. [71] used ovalbumin sensitised mice as an immune response model to study the immunoregulation effect of aqueous extract of honeysuckle. Water extract of honeysuckle could alleviate the inflammation of intestinal villi in allergic mice, reduce the aggregation and degranulation of mast cells, increase the ratio of intact mast cells in the lamina propria, reduce the release of histamine in the intestinal tract of allergic mice, reduce levels of interleukin-4 and ovalbumin, reduce the ratio of interleukin-4/interferon-γ in allergic mice and inhibit transcription levels of interleukin-12 in peripheral lymphoid tissue mononuclear cells.

4.6 Neuromodulation effects

The aroma of scented tea can relieve depression and reduce anxiety and also improve concentration, relieve physical stress and improve work efficiency. Studies have shown that inhaling the aroma of jasmine scented tea can improve the rate of simple mental arithmetic by 10% and alleviate tachycardia [72]. Kyoko et al. [73] showed that inhaling the aroma of jasmine scented tea for 5 min can significantly reduce heart rate, making people feel calm and energetic. Another study reported that the aroma of jasmine scented tea contained (R)-(−)-linalool, which plays a sedative role in human autonomic nervous activity and emotional state. Li et al. [29] conducted a study on the intervention effect of rose scented tea on postpartum depression and found that rose scented tea could reduce the Edinburgh Postpartum Depression Scale score in patients with postpartum depression and alleviate related symptoms to varying degrees. Subsequently, Zhai et al. [74] conducted a comparative study on rose scented tea and sweet orange essential oil, which has sedative effects. Inhalation of rose scented tea and sweet orange essential oil using aromatherapy lamps significantly reduced blood pressure and heart rate and rose scented tea was better at relieving the systolic blood pressure. Scented tea contains high amounts of volatile substances, which together form the unique aroma of scented tea. Among these, hydrocarbons, alcohols, esters and phenolic compounds are volatilised after brewing and heating the scented tea. These substances are absorbed by the capillaries of the lungs and then transported to the whole body via the blood, relieving the muscles and brain cells of the body.

5. Conclusions

China has established a refined tea production system and is a leader in research into scented tea ingredients. Scented tea is used medicinally and as a foodstuff and drink. The health benefits of scented tea on the human body are well established. Advances in human nutrition and increased interest in physical health have led to increased attention about the nutrition and health benefits of food. Studies have shown that the polyphenols and flavonoids present in scented tea promote human physical health, which keeps the market share of scented tea in China high.

However, the health benefits of scented tea should not be overstated. Scented tea is a health drink, not a drug, and it regulates but does not cure the human body. In addition, attention should be paid to the application of chemical fertilisers and pesticides in the cultivation of flowers and tea as pesticide residues in scented tea may seriously affect its quality and safety. Attention should be paid to the selection of raw materials used in the preparation of scented tea. Fresh, plump flowers and tea are used as raw materials and the flowers and tea are processed in strict accordance with the scenting process. Finally, the health benefits of scented tea are not achieved by a single substance, but the synergistic effects of multiple chemical components, which should be considered comprehensively when using scented tea.

Acknowledgements

This work was supported by the Yunnan Provincial Natural Science Foundation (Grant No. 202101AT070038), Yunnan Agricultural joint project (202101BD070001-105), China Scholarship Council, and, as well as the Yunnan Provincial Youth top talent project (Grant No. YNWR-QNBJ-2020-166), Natural science foundation of Yunnan Provincial department of education (2022Y553) and Middle-age Reserve Talents of Academic and Technical Leaders (2019HB026) and the 111 project (D21027).

Author contributions

Writing-original draft, Bowen Liu; supervision, Jun Zhang, review & editing, Guanben Du, Shuduan Deng and Xiaojian Zhou.

Author details

Bowen Liu, Jun Zhang*, Xiaojian Zhou, Shuduan Deng and Guanben Du
Yunnan Provincial Key Laboratory of Wood Adhesives and Glued Products,
Southwest Forestry University, Kunming, China

*Address all correspondence to: zj8101274@163.com

References

[1] Huang LF, Li Q, Han X, et al. Formation of sensory terminology and construction of flavor wheel of Chinese scented tea based on ancient scripts research. Aem Roducts Rocessing. 2022;**3**:62-65

[2] Xiao ZG, Zhu YW, Zhang XL. Research on the origin and development of jasmine tea. Tea Communication. 2021;**48**(1):173-176

[3] Bai LL, Liu Y. Evaluation and analysis of contemporary "medicinal tea" research. Chinese General Practice Nursing. 2020;**18**(33):4545-4548

[4] Jiang HY, Ma YX, Huang JF, et al. The research status of Jasmine tea health care efficacy and related health care products. Journal of Shanxi Agricultural University (Natural Science Edition). 2016;**36**(8):604-608

[5] Yu J, Yj G, Zhang Y, et al. Talking about the production and development of traditional Chinese medicine substitute tea. Diet Health. 2020;**7**(11):112

[6] Shen Q, Pan K, Si HQ, et al. Analysis on chemical components of new-type chloranthus Spicatus scented tea. Guizhou Agricultural Sciences. 2011;**39**(08):72-76

[7] Wang WW, Zhang JY, Wang W, et al. Development and utilization of caffeine in tea. China Tea. 2021;**43**(5):4

[8] Wu J, Wang C, Yu HC. Chemical constituents and pharmacological effect of lonicerae Japonicae flos. Chinese Journal of Experimental Traditional Medical Formulae. 2019;**25**(04):225-234

[9] Yasuyoshi M, Tomohiro SM, Kyohei A, et al. Anticancer effects of green tea and the nderlying molecular mechanisms in bladder cancer. Medicine. 2018;**5**(3):87

[10] Kong DD, Zhao YL, Wang YF, et al. Review on inhibition mechanism of tea polyphenols against tumor immune escape. Journal of Zhejiang University (Agriculture & Life Sciences). 2018;**44**(05):539-548

[11] Xie J, Zhao HY, Tian Y. Tumor cell apoptosis induced by EGCG in green tea and its mechanism: A research review. Modern Food Science & Technology. 2021;**37**(09):333-339

[12] Ma H, Ru X, Wang J, Zhao LM, et al. Study on the antioxidant capacity of four tea water extracts and tea polyphenols in vitro. Food Research and Development. 2019;**40**(08):65-70

[13] Chen MC, Zhu YJ, Wang JP, et al. Effect of jasmine tea scenting process on the inhibition activity of proliferation of cancer cell. Journal of Food Safety and Quality Inspection. 2019;**10**(13):4209-4216

[14] Yang YY, Wan XH, Liu YN, et al. Research progress on chemical constituents and pharmacological effects of Sedum sarmentosum. China Journal of Chinese Materia Medica. 2020;**45**(18):4341-4348

[15] Diego C, Menezes A, Garcia F, et al. Murraya paniculata (L.) (Orange Jasmine): Potential nutraceuticals with ameliorative effect in alloxan-induced diabetic rats. Phytotherapy Research: PTR. 2017;**31**(11):1747-1756

[16] Wang M, Jiang YL, Kuang XC, et al. Effects of jasmine and jasmine tea extracts on functions of mouse immune

cells. Chinese Journal of Pathophysiology. 2011;**27**(7):1428-1430

[17] Liu J, Yang JF. Primary studies on the anti-depression function of jasmine tea. Journal of Shanxi Agricultural University (Natural Science Edition). 2013;**33**(6):493-497

[18] Li ML, Xiao WJ, Gong ZH, et al. Scenting techniques of jasmine tea from broken green tea. Journal of Hunan Agricultural University. 2002;**28**(5):411-420

[19] Liu F, Wang Y, Li CH, et al. Research status and prospect of tea drying technology. Chinese Agricultural Science Bulletin. 2015;**31**(6):210-215

[20] Yuan ZY. Effect of sanzhu jiangfei decoction on blood-lipid, leptin and pancreatic lipase of experimental rats. Shandong Journal of Traditional Chinese Medicine. 2004;**23**(11):680-682

[21] Zhu QJ, Li H. The mechanism of losing weight of sanzhu jianfei decoction on alimentary obesity rats. China Journal of Chinese Medicine. 2014;**7**:1010-1011

[22] Xie XH, Xu L, Chen PX, et al. Research progress on technology for processing green teas with flowery aroma. Journal of Tea. 2022;**48**(1):20-24

[23] Hu Y, Du YP, Tian CJ, et al. A review of chemical components and their bioactivities from the genus lilium. Food Science. 2018;**39**(15):323-332

[24] Hu MM, Cai BC, Zhang ZJ, et al. Pharmacodynamics research of lilium brownii polysaccharide. Traditional Chinese Drug Research & Clinical Pharmacology. 2007;**18**(2):107-109

[25] Zhang J, Peng D, Chen K, et al. Research progress on the effect of lilium polysaccharide on immunity. Chinese Journal of Veterinary Parasitology. 2021;**29**(3):114-118

[26] Li CY, Wang W, Zhang LF, et al. Comparison of a kind of rose tea and other teas processing research. Academic Periodical of Farm Products Processing. 2021;**6**(41-42):47

[27] Zong NY, Zhang ZG. Research progress in the processing and exploitation edible roses. Aem Roducts Rocessing. 2017;**9**(44-46):52

[28] Yang CS, Lambert JD, Ju J, et al. Tea and cancer prevention: Molecular mechanisms and human relevance. Toxicology and Applied Pharmacology. 2007;**224**(3):265-273

[29] Li JZ, Wang HX, Zuo XL. A clinical trial of rose tea in treatment of postpartum depression. Maternal & Child Health Care Of China. 2010;**25**(34):5125-5127

[30] Luo L, Ye M, Lin J, et al. Research progress on composition and processing of Flos Lonicerae. Food & Machinery. 2022;**38**(4):228-233

[31] Miao S, Wan FC, Shen WJ, et al. Advances in application status of lonicera Japonica. Flos and its by-products in livestock and poultry. Chinese Journal of Animal Science. 2022;**58**(2):27-31

[32] Wan YY, Du WW, Chen JR, et al. Study on quantity-quality transfer from Lonicera Japonica Flos to standard decoction. Hebei Journal of Industrial Science & Technology. 2022;**39**(2):129-143

[33] Yan RH, Zhang YY, Guo YN, et al. Structural basis for the recognition of the 2019-nCoV by human ACE2. Science. 2020;**367**(6485):1444-1448

[34] Ge LL, Wan HQ, Tang SM, et al. Novel caffeoylquinic acid derivatives

from Lonicera japonica Thunb. flower buds exert pronounced anti-HBV activities. RSC Advances. 2018;**8**(62):35374-35385

[35] Zhu JL, Li H, Qin Y, et al. Preparation of nano silver from honeysuckle extracts and its antibacterial properties for fabric. Journal of Dalian Dalian Polytechnic University. 2021;**40**(5):339-344

[36] Yang CS, Maliakal P, Meng X. Inhibition of carcinogenesis by tea. Annual Review of Pharmacology and Toxicology. 2002;**42**:25-54

[37] Chen TT, Yang CS. Biological fates of tea polyphenols and their interactions with microbiota in the gastrointestinal tract: implications on health effects. Critical reviews in food science and nutrition. 2020;**60**(16):2691-2709

[38] Zhang ZL, Hao XL, Dai SJ, et al. Study on extraction of flavonoids from jasmine tea and their antimicrobial activities. Guangzhou Chemical Industry. 2020;**48**(6):93-95

[39] Li SZ. Compendium of Materia Medica. Beijing: People's Medical Publishing House; 1982

[40] Feng SL, He L, Wang M, et al. Studies on the chemical constituents of flower of david lily. China Journal Of Chinese Materia Medica. 1994;**10**(611-612):639

[41] Zhou QX, Yue SM. Analysis of the research status of Osmanthus fragrans Lour in chemical constituents and pharmacological actions based on literature. Journal Of Henan University(Medical Science). 2013;**32**(2):139-142

[42] Wang M, Liu F, Lin CH, et al. Impacts of different drying methods on antioxidant activity and chemical ingredients of honeysuckle by chemiluminescence detection. Shandong Science. 2013;**26**(2):56-65

[43] Li YS. Landscape characteristics and exploitation value of rosa rugosa. Journal Of Beijing Agricultural Vocation College. 2010;**24**(6):25-28

[44] Wu WJ, Zhao ZH, Zhang Y, et al. Research progress in LC-MS technology for the analysis of chemical composition from medicine and food dual purposes plants. Science and Technology of Food Industry. 2016;**37**(19):366-371

[45] Lin PF, Jia XZ, Qi Y, et al. Advances in study on phenolic acids. Guangdong Chemical Industry. 2017;**44**(1):50-52

[46] Song YL, Wang HM, Ni FY, et al. Study on anti-inflammatory activities of phenolic acids from Lonicerae Japonicae Flos. Chinese Traditional and Herbal Drugs. 2015;**46**(4):490-495

[47] Zhang ZB, Shen HK, Sun YF, et al. Studied on phenolic acids extracting of Lonicera japonica Thunb. and its antimicrobial Effect. Chinese Journal of Ethnomedicine and Ethnopharmacy. 2019;**28**(16):27-29

[48] Liu ZH, Lai XL, Liu HX. Discussion on the action mechanism of Radix Astragali seu Hedysar-Herba Pogostemonis-Flos Lonicerae in the prevention of COVID-19 based on network pharmacology. Global Traditional Chinese Medicine. 2021;**14**(2):215-224

[49] Cong T, Zhao L, Li Z, et al. The effects of three kind of jasmine tea on nutritional physiological functions of growing rats. Modern Preventive Medicine. 2011;**38**(03):456-460

[50] Zhou HJ, Li TZ, Li B. Identification of antioxidant components and

tyrosinase specific inhibitors from osmanthus fragrans flower by using online UPLC-ABTS+•-assay and UF-LC-MS technology. Science and Technology of Food Industry. 2022;**43**(7):67-79

[51] Bao QL, Wang D, Lu KQ, et al. Study on the antioxidative activities of flavonoids from osmanthus fragrans in vivo and in vitro. Food Research and Development. 2018;**39**(21):14-20

[52] Chen W, Zhang J, Chang P, et al. Effect of rose extract on tail suspension test and antioxidant capacity in stressed mice. Science and Technology of Food Industry. 2012;**1**:376-378

[53] Liu J, Zhao QN, Zeng QQ. Advances in chemical constituents and pharmacological activities of roses. Food and Drug. 2019;**21**(4):328-332

[54] Liao L, Lu L, Yang C, et al. Bioinformatics and molecular docking analysis of the effect of honeysuckle on gene expression in lung cancer. Journal of Kunming University of Science and Technology(Natural Science Edition). 2022;**47**(1):87-99

[55] Yan BF, Liu J, Liu SJ, et al. Effects of apoptosis induced by methanolic extract of Rosa rugosa Thunb. in prostate cancer PC-3 cells based upon ROS/PI3K/Akt/mTOR signaling pathway. Chinese Journal of Hospital Pharmacy. 2021;**41**(19):1987-1992

[56] Iwai K, Kishimoto N, Kakino Y, et al. In vitro antioxidative effects and tyrosinase inhibitory activities of seven hydroxycinnamoyl derivatives in green coffee beans. Journal of Agricultural and Food Chemistry. 2004;**52**(15):4893-4898

[57] Mijangos-Ramos IF, Zapata-Estrella HE, Ruiz-Vargas JA, et al. Bioactive dicaffeoylquinic acid derivatives from the root extract of Calea urticifolia. Revista Brasileira de Farmacognosia. 2018;**28**(3):339-343

[58] Li XC, Li K, Xie H, et al. Antioxidant and cytoprotective effects of the Di-O-caffeoylquinic acid family: The mechanism, structure-activity relationship, and conformational effect. Molecules. 2018;**23**(1):222

[59] Kawabata K, Yamamoto T, Hara A, et al. Modifying effects of ferulic acid on azoxymethane-induced colon carcinogenesis in F344 rats. Cancer Letters. 2000;**157**(1):15-21

[60] Xie ZF, Guo ZY, Wang Y, et al. Protocatechuic acid inhibits the growth of ovarian cancer cells by inducing apoptosis and autophagy. Phytotherapy Research. 2018;**32**(11):2256-2263

[61] Wu ZH, Cheng WM, Zhang ZY, et al. Chemical constituents of ethyl acetate fractions of Inonotus obliquus and in vitro antitumor activity. Journal of Anhui Medical University. 2018;**53**(11):1757-1761

[62] Chen WZ. Synthesis and anti-tumor activity of NO donor caffeic acid derivatives. Journal of Suzhou University. 2020;**35**(9):75-78

[63] Huang S, Wang LL, Xue NN, et al. Chlorogenic acid effectively treats cancers through induction of cancer cell differentiation. Theranostics. 2019;**9**(23):6745-6763

[64] Lin JX, Huang JF, Yan TY, et al. Research progress on hypoglycemic and hypolipidemic effects of jasmine tea. Tea Communication. 2021;**48**(3):405-414

[65] Cao NF, Li YY, Cui WH, et al. α-glucosidase inhibitory activity of Osmanthus fragrans Lour. (Wanyingui,Yaotiaoshunv and

Guifeihong). Journal Of Henan University(Medical Science). 2010;**29**(1):21-23

[66] Zhu WQ, Ren HS, Zheng YY, et al. Research progress in functional components and bioactivity of honeysuckle. Science and Technology of Food Industry. 2021;**42**(13):412-426

[67] Tian YH, Feng YL, Wang XY, et al. Research progress on quality evaluation of chemical components and edible and medicinal use of rosa rugosa. Quality Safety Inspection and Testing. 2022;**32**(2):43-68

[68] Lan W, Wang Y, Hao YW, et al. Effects of Uygur Medicine Branchlets roses extracts on blood glucose and glucose tolerance in diabetes mice induced by alloxan. Drug Evaluation Research. 2017;**40**(4):492-495

[69] Zhu Q, Zeng L, Li GX, et al. Preliminary study on the mechanism of water extraction from honeysuckle total flavonoids on blood lipids in hyperlipidemic mice. China Preventive Medicine. 2020;**21**(7):737-743

[70] Lin PG, Pan WQ, Luo WG, et al. Study on the prevention of acute renal failure in mice by jasmine tea and compound tea. Journal of Air Force Medical College. 1994;**2**:15-17

[71] Li F, Li H. Immunoregulatory effects of the Lonicera aquatic extract in the ovalbulmin-sensitized BALB/c mice. Chinese Journal of Pediatrics. 2005;**43**(11):852-857

[72] Yang QT, Yang QB. Research progress on health efficacy of jasmine tea. Fujian Tea. 2020;**42**(9):3-5

[73] Kuroda K, Inoue N, Ito Y, et al. Sedative effects of the jasmine tea odor and (R)-(−)-linalool, one of its major odor components, on autonomic nerve activity and mood states. European Journal of Applied Physiology. 2005;**95**:107-114

[74] Zhai XL, Yu YW, Wu YY, et al. Research and development of aromatherapy. Flavour Fragrance Cosmetics. 2011;**6**:45-50

Chapter 6

GABA-enriched Oolong Tea: Reducing Stress in a Student Cohort May Involve More than Just GABA

Tina Hinton, Kong M. Li, Vincent Viengkhou, Sin Yoo Kam, Sandra Kindaro, Herbert F. Jelinek, Slade Matthews and Graham A.R. Johnston

Abstract

We have previously shown that the consumption of GABA-enriched oolong tea is effective in reducing stress in a student cohort. However, key constituent content has not been previously investigated, especially as applied to a standard cup of tea. Further, it has not been substantiated whether it is the suggested GABA content or other constituents that lead to these observed changes in stress behaviour. Using reverse-phase HPLC, we determined the actual content of four chemicals known to influence stress in 200 mL cups of regular or GABA-enriched oolong tea brewed to manufacturer's instructions. We found eight times as much γ-aminobutyric acid (GABA) and 1.5 times as much caffeine in GABA-enriched oolong tea as in regular oolong tea. In contrast, there was 10 times less epigallocatechin gallate (EGCG), and half as much theanine in the GABA-enriched tea. Thus, there are changes in multiple constituents in GABA-enriched oolong tea that may contribute to the biological effects we observed in students consuming these teas.

Keywords: GABA, theanine, epigallocatechin gallate, caffeine, tea, stress, HPLC

1. Introduction

We have previously shown that consumption of GABA-enriched oolong tea is effective in reducing stress and improving cardiac rhythm in a university student cohort [1]. As constituents other than GABA are known to influence stress, we have quantified three other key chemicals in oolong tea known to influence stress: the methylxanthine caffeine, the flavonoid epigallocatechin gallate (EGCG) and the amino acid theanine in addition to GABA. The chemical structures of these constituents are shown in **Figure 1**. The aim of the current study was to quantify, using HPLC, the concentrations of these constituents in 200 mL cups of regular oolong and GABA-enriched oolong tea as prepared according to manufacturer's specifications and consumed by the students.

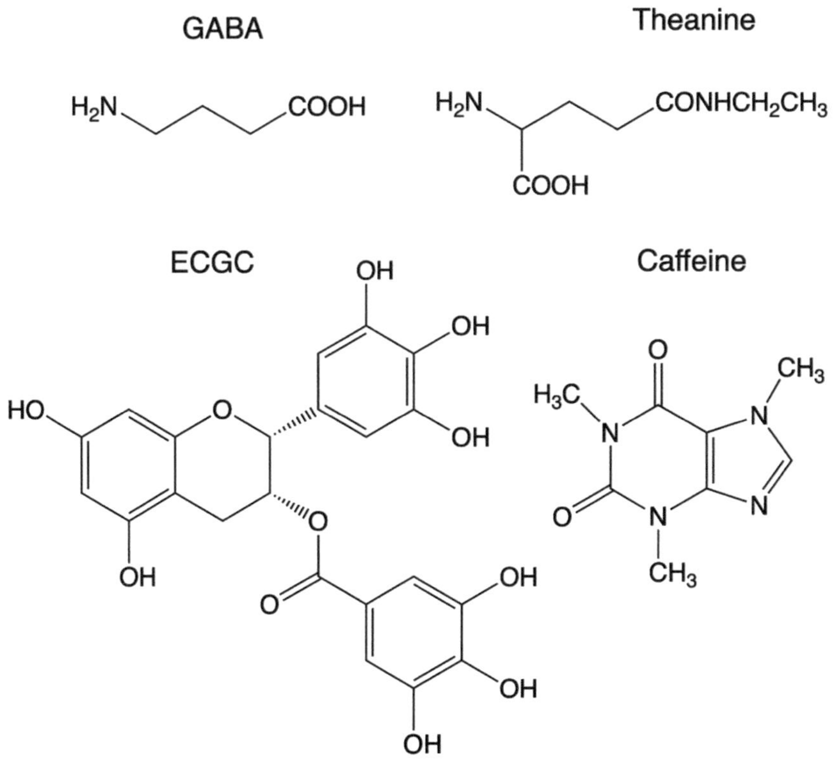

Figure 1.
Chemical structures of four neuroactive constituents found in regular oolong and GABA-enriched oolong teas.

GABA is the major inhibitory neurotransmitter in the brain [2] and plays a pivotal role in stress as well as modulating autonomic and cardiovascular function centrally and peripherally. GABA-enriched foods and GABA in single oral administration have been shown to reduce stress as measured through heart rate variability, heart rate, and other stress-related biomarkers and psychological tests. Hence, GABA content in tea has been enhanced to produce an improved therapeutically useful beverage for consumption [3]. GABA-enriched tea is obtained by incubation of tea under anaerobic conditions, or cycling under aerobic and anaerobic conditions, which has been shown to accumulate GABA to produce a tea with concentrations of GABA >150 mg/100 g tea [4–9].

The possible roles for other oolong tea constituents of oolong tea, such as EGCG, theanine and caffeine, may then also relate to their interaction with GABA. There are several known mechanisms of action to explain the effects of caffeine in oolong tea in addition to its stimulant effect [10]. The most prominent is that it is a potent adenosine receptor antagonist, and it has also been shown to potentiate GABA release via its effect on A_1 adenosine receptors [11].

EGCG may mediate some of its stress-reducing effects via interaction with the GABAergic system [12–15]. EGCG is readily incorporated into the brain following intragastric administration in mice [14], and has shown stress-reducing, anxiolytic and sedative properties in a number of animal models [12, 13, 15]. EGCG has also been found to be a biphasic modulator of $GABA_A$ receptors, at low doses enhancing diazepam action at recombinant $GABA_A$ receptors expressed in *Xenopus* oocytes [16].

Although the action of theanine is not well understood [17, 18], it has been proposed to contribute to the relaxation experienced following tea consumption. For example, an oral 200 mg dose of theanine was also shown to increase α-brain waves in the occipital and parietal cortices of human subjects, indicative of a relaxation effect [17]. While one study showed it to increase GABA release [19], theanine does not appear to impact behaviours mediated by the GABAergic system in animal models [19–21]. Instead, theanine may mediate its effects through modulation of other transmitter systems including dopamine [18, 22] and glycine [22].

The aim of the current study was to quantify, using HPLC, the concentrations of GABA, EGCG, caffeine and theanine in 200 mL cups of regular oolong and GABA-enriched oolong tea as prepared according to manufacturer's specifications and consumed by the students.

2. Materials and methods

2.1 HPLC sample preparation and analysis

Golden Wulong (regular Oolong tea) and Organic GABA Body and Mind tea (GABA-enriched Oolong tea) both originated from Taiwan and were purchased from www.teas.com.au. Standard cups of each oolong tea were prepared and analysed to quantify both the differences in active constituent content between the teas and also the consistency of GABA, theanine, caffeine and EGCG extraction between separate brews of the same tea. Teas were prepared in accordance with manufacturer's instructions for consumption, by the addition of 5 g tea to 200 mL of 90°C deionised Milli-Q water (dH_2O) and infused for 10 min.

Samples (20 mg) of the authentic standard compounds, GABA (RBI; Natick, MA, U.S.A.), theanine (Tocris; Ballwin, MO, U.S.A.), caffeine (Sigma, St. Louis, MO, U.S.A.) and EGCG (Sigma, St. Louis, MO, U.S.A.), were weighed accurately and added to a 100 mL volumetric flask before being dissolved in 12.5% acetonitrile, yielding final stock solutions of 200 μg/mL. Standard solutions in the range of 5.0–200 μg/mL were made by diluting the stock solution with 12.5% acetonitrile directly before each run. The standard solutions were filtered through 0.45 μm, 13 mm diameter HPLC nylon syringe filters (Grace Davison Discovery Science; Deerfield, IL, U.S.A.). Analysis was via reverse-phase HPLC using a Varian ProStar 210 solvent delivery system coupled to a Varian autosampler model 410 with cooling tray set at 4°C, Degassit degasser (Varian Inc.; Walnut Creek, CA, U.S.A.). Data were collected and analysed using Varian Star Chromatography Workstation, Interactive Graphic, System Control and Method Builder version 6.30 (Varian Inc.).

2.2 GABA and theanine measurements

GABA and theanine were determined using pre-column derivatisation of standards and tea samples at the same time before each run for detection of amino acids. Immediately prior to derivatisation, 50 μL tea samples were mixed with 50 μL 0.2 M borate buffer (pH 8.5). To derivatise the amino acids, 100 μL 15.5 mM 9-fluorenylmethyloxycarbonyl chloride (FMOC-Cl) was added and allowed to react for 1 min before addition of 60 μL cleavage reagent (0.5 M hydroxylamine hydrochloride: 1.7 M sodium hydroxide: water) to remove excess FMOC-Cl which can interfere with amino acid separation. The reaction was stopped after three minutes with 100 μL quenching reagent (1:4 glacial acetic acid: acetonitrile). Each sample was then diluted 1:3 in water and filtered through a 0.45 µm HPLC nylon syringe filter (13 mm diameter). All samples were stored at 4 °C and analysed within 24 hours.

For amino acid detection, a Shimadzu RF-10A$_{XL}$ spectrofluorometric detector (excitation 263 nm; emission 313 nm) with a Varian Microsorb-MV 100 C18, 5 µm, 250 × 4.6 mm column maintained at room temperature were used.

2.3 Caffeine and EGCG measurements

For caffeine and EGCG quantification, samples were centrifuged at 2,500 g for 10 mins, a 1:2.5 dilution was made using 12.5% acetonitrile, and then samples were filtered through 0.45 µm, 13 mm diameter HPLC nylon syringe filters. All samples were stored at 4°C for no greater than 24 hours prior to performing HPLC. For caffeine and EGCG measurement, a Kinetex 5u XB-C18 (5 µm, 150 × 4.6 mm) column maintained at room temperature was used. Detection was via analysis at UV wavelength 254 nm.

2.4 Gradient elution

All chromatographic experiments were performed using gradient elution. For GABA and theanine, optimised mobile phase A consisted of 2 M ammonium phosphate buffer (pH 6.7), methanol and water (0.75:15:84.25). Mobile Phase B was acetonitrile and water (90:10). For caffeine and EGCG, the composition of the optimised mobile phase A was water/acetonitrile/formic acid (94.7/4.3/1) and mobile phase B was water/acetonitrile/formic acid (49.5/49.5/1). Each mobile phase was filtered through a 0.45 µm Teflon membrane filter under vacuum prior to use. The flow rate was 1.0 mL/min.

The gradient elution profile for GABA and theanine was 0 min 12% B, 5 min 30% B, 20 min 34% B and 22–27 min 99% B. The gradient elution profile for caffeine and EGCG was 0 min 1% B, 10 min 35% B, 13.3 min 90% B, 19.5 min 90% B, 21 min 1% B and 26 min 1% B. The injection volume was 5 µL and the detection wavelength was set at 254 nm. GABA, theanine, caffeine and EGCG were identified by comparison of the retention time of peaks produced by the tea sample against that of the respective GABA, theanine, caffeine and EGCG standards.

2.5 Method validation

Calibration curves were constructed from duplicate analyses of GABA and theanine standards at 1.2, 2.4, 4.8, 7.2, 9.6 and 12.0 µM, and triplicate analyses of caffeine and EGCG standards at 5, 50, 100, 160 and 200 µM. To evaluate the intraday and interday precision, 96 µM GABA and theanine standards were analysed in duplicate of two consecutive days, 50 µM caffeine and 160 µM EGCG standards were analysed in triplicate on three consecutive days, and coefficients of variation (CV) for the retention time and peak area were calculated. Accuracy was assessed using a recovery test of spiked samples with 50 µM of each of GABA, theanine, caffeine and EGCG. Recoveries were calculated comparing the obtained amounts with those added using the formula: recovery (%) = [(concentration found – endogenous concentration) / 50] × 100% (Zhao *et al.*, 2011). Validation of GABA, theanine, caffeine and EGCG peak identification in the samples was conducted by comparing the retention time of the peak of increased size in the spiked to the unspiked samples.

3. Results

3.1 HPLC method validation

Mean retention times of the standards were: GABA 14.05 min; theanine 13.15 min; caffeine 8.65 min; and EGCG 11.32 min. Consistent retention times were also observed for both regular oolong tea (GABA 14.08 min; theanine 13.19 min; caffeine 8.46 min; and EGCG 11.21 min) and GABA-enriched oolong tea (GABA 14.01 min; theanine 13.11 min; caffeine 8.39 min; and EGCG 11.13 min). The calibration curves for quantified constituents obtained from the duplicate and triplicate standards exhibited linear correlation coefficients (r^2) of 0.991 for GABA, 0.996 for theanine, 0.992 for caffeine, and 0.998 for EGCG. Intraday CVs of peak area and retention time were GABA 1.61%; theanine 0.01%; caffeine 1.03%; and EGCG 0.06%. Interday CVs were GABA 5.41%; theanine 0.01%; caffeine 2.45%; and EGCG 0.01%. The spiked samples demonstrated mean recoveries of 100.33 ± 28.40% (range: 87–134%) for GABA and theanine, and 104.64 ± 19.07% for caffeine and EGCG.

3.2 GABA, theanine, caffeine and EGCG content in a cup of tea

Two separate brews of each tea were analysed in duplicate for GABA and theanine, and three separate brews were analysed in triplicate for caffeine and EGCG in order to determine both the difference in constituent content between the teas and also the consistency of constituent content between separate brews of the same tea. Given the greater degree of variability encountered with the measurement of the caffeine and EGCG content in different brews, triplicate measurements were undertaken. The relative amounts of GABA, theanine, caffeine and EGCG and differences in constituent content between the two types of tea are shown in **Table 1** expressed as mg per 200 mL of brewed tea from 5 g of dry tea leaf. Good reproducibility in the extraction of constituents was demonstrated with our preparation protocol. Both teas showed consistent quantified constituent content between separate brews of the same tea.

Representative reverse-phase HPLC chromatograms are shown in **Figures 2** and **3**.

Constituent (mg/100 g)	Regular tea				GABA-enriched tea			
	Brew 1	Brew 2	Brew 3	Average	Brew 1	Brew 2	Brew 3	Average
GABA	5.00	5.00		5.00	40.4	40.0		40.2
Theanine	163	166		165	82.8	82.0		82.4
Caffeine	300	252	250	267	457	368	383	402
EGCG	377	355	338	356	1.80	3.60	2.40	2.60

Data are expressed in mg per 100 g of dry tea leaf.

Table 1.
Amount of GABA, theanine, caffeine and EGCG in separate brews of oolong tea.

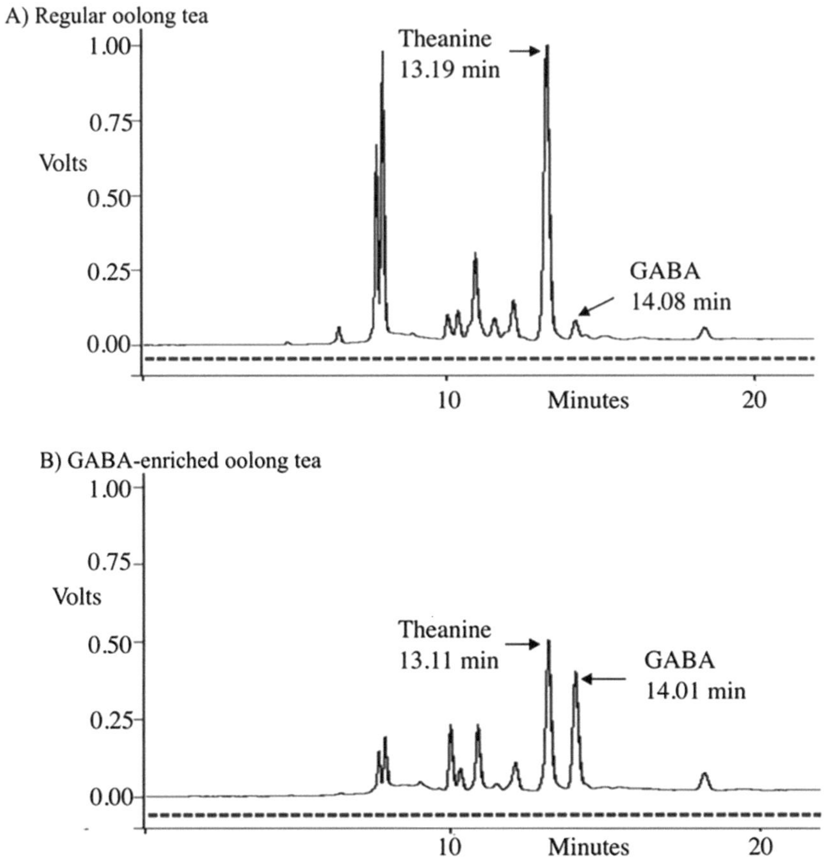

Figure 2.
Representative reverse-phase HPLC chromatograms of GABA and theanine in (A) regular oolong, and (B) GABA-enriched oolong teas.

4. Discussion

The advantage of our study is that four active constituents of tea were measured using HPLC in one tea type (oolong) and changes relative to GABA-enrichment were documented. Further, our method of sample preparation was appropriate for determining constituent content in a cup of tea prepared according to usual consumption practices and in our studies of effects on a student cohort. In future, testing these constituents across a range of commercially available products would be valuable for a wider comparison of different tea types. Choice of oolong tea for the current study was based on mid-range fermentation. Analysis of constituents of GABA-enriched green or black teas will likely yield differing results.

Previous studies using HPLC have determined GABA to be present to varying extents in commercially prepared GABA-enriched teas, including 1560 mg/100 g [9]; 19 mg/100 g [6] and 272 mg/100 g [4]. The type of tea according to the degree of oxidation (e.g., oolong, black) was not specified in these studies. On the other hand, GABA concentration in freshly prepared GABA tea has been measured at between 30 and 700 mg/100 g (average 275 mg/100 g) using HPLC, with concentrations dependent on the method of preparation (aerobic vs anaerobic cycling, or both), and plant

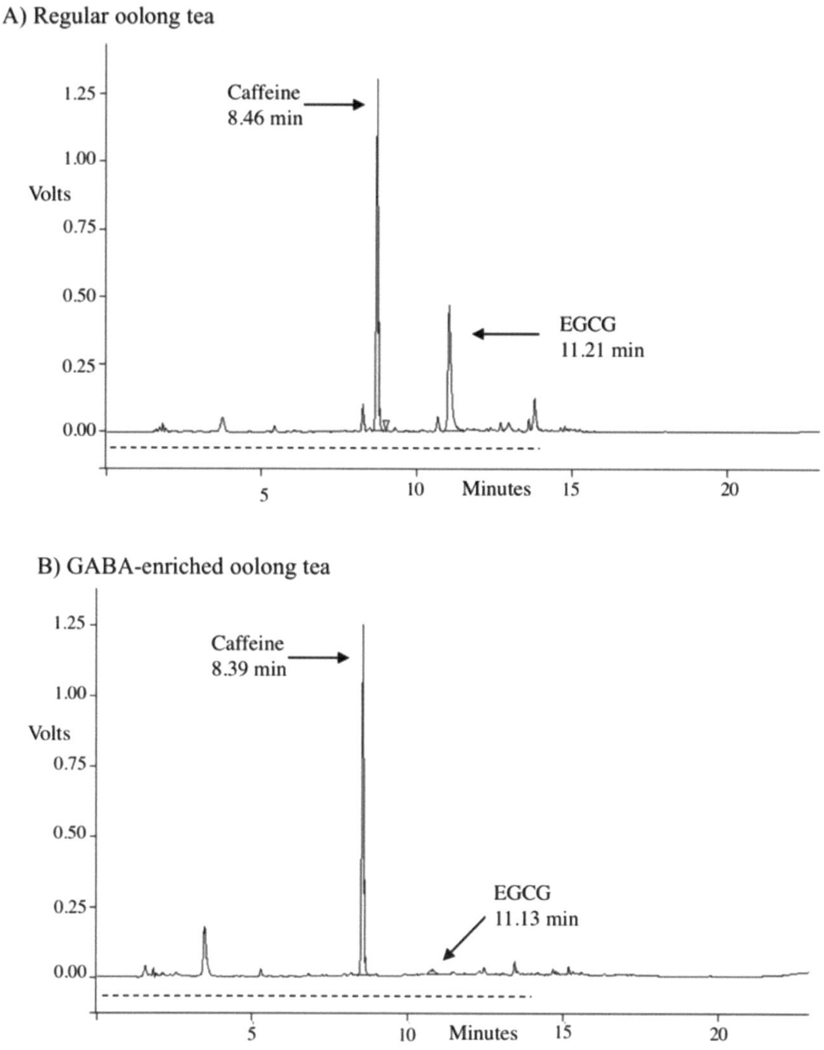

Figure 3.
Representative reverse-phase HPLC chromatograms of caffeine and EGCG in (A) regular oolong, and (B) GABA-enriched oolong teas.

part used (leaves, buds or stem) [5, 7, 8, 23, 24]. These reported results compare with our finding of 40.2 mg GABA/100 g GABA-enriched oolong tea.

In non-GABA enriched (i.e., regular) teas, GABA quantities have been measured using HPLC, Zhao et al. [9] found the concentration of GABA in teas differed according to tea type. Relative concentrations from greatest to least were white (50.5 mg/100 g) > black (31.1–41.5 mg/100 g) > green (13.8–33.9 mg/100 g) > oolong (14.8–20.7 mg/100 g). On the other hand, Syu and colleagues [6] found the GABA content of different teas to be green (19.6–105 mg/100 g) equal to oolong (10–101 mg/100 g) > black (34–55 mg/100 g). In contrast to our findings of 5 mg GABA/100 g regular oolong tea, others have shown, on average, higher GABA concentrations in commercially prepared regular oolong teas.

The differences between GABA content determined in our study and findings from previous investigations may be explained by the fact that our teas were prepared according to manufacturer's instructions using simple aqueous extraction, as in making a cup of tea, without repeated extractions using different solvents and drying down to increase yield. In this way, we provide a realistic estimation of the concentration of GABA that one may encounter in a commonly prepared cup of tea.

Like GABA, theanine content measured across a range of commercial tea types is found to vary in concentration, and even within the different tea types, there is significant variation [6, 25, 26]. For example, commercially prepared white teas measured between 53 and 3337 mg theanine/100 g w/w [25] while oolong teas ranged from 85 to 282 mg/100 g [25], averaging 101 mg/100 g [6]. Our findings of 163.2 mg/100 g of theanine in a cup of regular oolong tea are in keeping with these previous studies. One study that prepared tea for analysis similar to the method used in the present investigation (brewing for a specified period of time in 200 mL water) found a standard (200 mL) cup of black tea contained 24.2 mg L-theanine, white tea contained 11.5 mg, while a cup of green tea contained the least theanine at 7.9 mg [27]. These values are lower than those that we report and may be related to the type of tea tested. Oolong tea was not investigated by Keenan and colleagues [27].

Syu and colleagues [6] measured theanine content in GABA-enriched tea and found it occurred in a higher concentration (198 mg/100 g) than regular teas on average. This contrasts with our finding that GABA-enriched tea measured half the theanine concentration (82.4 mg/100 g) of the regular oolong tea. On the other hand, Wang et al., [8] and Tsushida and Murai [7] found that GABA enrichment did not substantially alter theanine concentration compared to non-enriched teas. Moreover, theanine content in black teas was shown to be equivalent to green and oolong teas [25–27], therefore it appears to remain unaffected by oxidation.

Zuo [28] found caffeine concentrations were fairly stable across different commercial teas tested, including green (up to 99 mg/ 100 g), oolong (37–121 mg/100 g) and black (43 mg/100 g) teas. Roughly equivalent amounts of caffeine were also found across different teas [29–31]. Caffeine constituted 3.62% w/w of white tea, ~2.40% w/w of green teas tested (0.77–3.35% w/w), 2.77% w/w of oolong tea, and ~2.90% w/w of black teas (2.41–3.69% w/w) [29–31].

Compared with previous studies, we show higher concentrations of caffeine in the teas we tested: 267 mg/100 g dried tea leaf in regular oolong tea and 402 mg/100 g in GABA-enriched oolong tea. These differences in concentration may be explained by the method of tea sample preparation for HPLC analysis. Zuo [28] extracted tea samples in methanol and HCl then further diluted samples in water, focusing on efficient extraction. Wang and colleagues [8] dried samples, infused them in 80°C water for 20 minutes, while we infused tea samples directly in 90°C water for 10 minutes in accordance with manufacturer's instructions for consumption.

Caffeine content has previously been shown to be relatively unaffected by the cycling fermentation process involved in creating GABA-enriched tea, with no difference between freshly prepared green (3.2 mg/100 g) and GABA-enriched (3.3 mg/100 g) [8] However, we found variation in caffeine content in GABA-enriched compared with regular oolong tea.

Our findings show a lower concentration of EGCG (356 mg/100 g) in regular oolong tea compared to some previous studies, and levels near the lower limit of detection in GABA-enriched oolong tea (2.6 mg/100 g). For example, Tang and colleagues [32] found that EGCG varied between 2070 mg/100 g and 3670 mg/100 g across commercially prepared oolong teas tested. This may be due to sample preparation as well as tea source. Tang et al., [32] extracted samples with 10 mL tetrahydrofuran at 30 °C for 30 minutes, followed by 10 mL methanol:acetic acid:water

(50:3.7:46.3, *v/v/v*) mixture at 30 °C for 30 minutes to obtain all soluble components. While this sample preparation technique may be more rigorous in extraction of different constituents, it does not represent common consumption practices. Thus, our findings provide a more realistic estimate of EGCG concentrations consumed in a cup of tea. The significant reduction in EGCG content in GABA-enriched compared with regular oolong tea observed in our study likely arose through the additional fermentation process required to increase GABA content in the tea.

There are many ways of increasing the levels of GABA in food and beverages. There is a wide range of GABA-enriched fermented food products [33], lactic acid fermented green tea being an example [34]. The GABA content of mulberry leave powder as a potential functional food ingredient has been increased by sodium glutamate immersion, cold shock and anoxia [35]. A different approach is being used in tomatoes, with CRISPR/Cas9 gene editing technology used to selectively increase GABA levels by deleting the autoinhibitory domain of the enzyme that converts glutamate to GABA [36]. GABA levels in such gene-edited tomatoes increased by 11- to 18-fold accompanied by a drastic reduction in glutamate and aspartate levels. Sales of these tomatoes were launched onto the Japanese market in 2021[37]. Such gene editing technology can be applied to annual crops like tomatoes but would be difficult to readily apply to tea.

In conclusion, teas contain a range of bioactive constituents including GABA, theanine, EGCG and caffeine. GABA-enriched oolong tea was shown to have 8 times more GABA than regular oolong tea, although the quantity may not be sufficient alone to account for the stress-reducing effects of this GABA-enriched tea. It is very likely that additional constituents measured here contribute to the purported relaxant effects of GABA-enriched tea, possibly via interaction with the GABAergic system. The differences in GABA, theanine, caffeine and EGCG content between GABA-enriched and regular oolong teas demonstrated here may arise through the additional fermentation process required to enrich GABA content in the tea. In particular, the increase in the amount of caffeine may be significant.

Acknowledgements

The authors thank Mr Thomas Santa of School of Medical Sciences (Pharmacology), The University of Sydney, for his expert help with the HPLC.

Author details

Tina Hinton[1], Kong M. Li[1], Vincent Viengkhou[2], Sin Yoo Kam[2], Sandra Kindaro[2], Herbert F. Jelinek[3], Slade Matthews[1] and Graham A.R. Johnston[1*]

1 Sydney Pharmacy School (Pharmacology), The University of Sydney, Australia

2 School of Medical Sciences (Pharmacology), The University of Sydney, Australia

3 Department of Biomedical Engineering, Healthcare Innovation Center and Center for Biotechnology, Khalifa University, Abu Dhabi, United Arab Emirates

*Address all correspondence to: graham.johnston@sydney.edu.au

References

[1] Hinton T, Jelinek HF, Viengkhou V, Johnston GAR, Matthews S. Effect of GABA-fortified oolong tea on reducing stress in a University Student Cohort. Frontiers in Nutrition. 2019;**6**:27

[2] Hinton T, Johnston GAR. GABA, the major inhibitory neurotransmitter in the brain. Reference Module in Biomedical Sciences. 2018;**2018**:1

[3] Hinton T, Johnston GAR. GABA-enriched teas as neuro-nutraceuticals. Neurochemistry International. 2020;**141**:104895. DOI: 10.1016/j.neuint.2020.104895

[4] Huang Y, Zheng H, Liu X, Wang X. Studies of the variation of GABA and Glu in Gabaron tea process. Food Science. 2005;**26**:117-120

[5] Sawai Y, Konomi K, Odaka Y, Yoshitomi H, Yamaguchi Y, Miyama D. Contents of γ-aminobutyric acid in stem of anaerobic incubated tea shoot [Japanese]. Journal of the Japanese Society for Food Science & Technology Nippon Shokuhin Kagaku Kogaku Kaishi. 1999;**46**(4):274-277

[6] Syu KY, Lin CL, Huang HC, Lin JK. Determination of theanine, GABA, and other amino acids in green, oolong, black, and Pu-erh teas with dabsylation and high-performance liquid chromatography. Journal of Agricultural and Food Chemistry. 2008;**56**(17):7637-7643. DOI: 10.1021/jf801795m

[7] Tsushida T, Murai T, Omori M, Okamoto J. Production of a new type tea containing a high-level of γ-aminobutyric-acid. Nippon Nogeikagaku Kaishi-J Jpn Soc Biosci Biotechol Agrochem. 1987;**61**(7):817-822

[8] Wang HF, Tsai YS, Lin ML, Ou AS-m. Comparison of bioactive components in GABA tea and green tea produced in Taiwan. Food Chemistry. 2006;**96**(4):648-653. DOI: 10.1016/j.foodchem.2005.02.046

[9] Zhao M, Ma Y, Wei ZZ, Yuan WX, Li YL, Zhang CH, et al. Determination and comparison of gamma-aminobutyric acid (GABA) content in pu-erh and other types of Chinese tea. Journal of Agricultural and Food Chemistry. 2011;**59**(8):3641-3648. DOI: 10.1021/jf104601v

[10] Hindmarch I, Rigney U, Stanley N, Quinlan P, Rycroft J, Lane J. A naturalistic investigation of the effects of day-long consumption of tea, coffee and water on alertness, sleep onset and sleep quality. Psychopharmacology. 2000;**149**(3):203-216. DOI: 10.1007/s002130000383

[11] Ferreira DD, Stutz B, de Mello FG, Reis RA, Kubrusly RC. Caffeine potentiates the release of GABA mediated by NMDA receptor activation: Involvement of A1 adenosine receptors. Neuroscience. 2014;**281**:208-215. DOI: 10.1016/j.neuroscience.2014.09.060

[12] Adachi N, Tomonaga S, Tachibana T, Denbow DM, Furuse M. (-)-Epigallocatechin gallate attenuates acute stress responses through GABAergic system in the brain. European Journal of Pharmacology. 2006;**531**(1-3):171-175. DOI: 10.1016/j.ejphar.2005.12.024

[13] Park K-S, Han J-Y, Moon D-C, Hong JT, Oh K-W. (–)-Epigallocatechin-3-O-Gallate augments pentobarbital-induced sleeping behaviors through Cl– channel activation. Journal of

Medicinal Food. 2011;**14**(11):1456-1462. DOI: 10.1089/jmf.2010.1529

[14] Suganuma M, Okabe S, Oniyama M, Tada Y, Ito H, Fujiki H. Wide distribution of H-3 (-)-epigallocatechin gallate, a cancer preventive tea polyphenol, in mouse tissue. Carcinogenesis. 1998;**19**(10):1771-1776. DOI: 10.1093/carcin/19.10.1771

[15] Vignes M, Maurice T, Lante F, Nedjar M, Thethi K, Guiramand J, et al. Anxiolytic properties of green tea polyphenol (-)-epigallocatechin gallate (EGCG). Brain Research. 2006;**1110**(1):102-115. DOI: 10.1016/j.brainres.2006.06.062

[16] Campbell EL, Chebib M, Johnston GAR. The dietary flavonoids apigenin and (-)-epigallocatechin gallate enhance the positive modulation by diazepam of the activation by GABA of recombinant GABA(A) receptors. Biochemical Pharmacology. 2004;**68**(8):1631-1638. DOI: 10.1016/j.bcp.2004.07.022

[17] Juneja LR, Chu D-C, Okubo T, Nagato Y, Yokogoshi H. Corrigendum to "L-theanine—a unique amino acid of green tea and its relaxation effect in humans". Trends in Food Science Technology. 1999;**10**(12):425

[18] Yokogoshi H, Kobayashi M, Mochizuki M, Terashima T. Effect of theanine, r-glutamylethylamide, on brain monoamines and striatal dopamine release in conscious rats. Neurochemical Research. 1998;**23**(5):667-673. DOI: 10.1023/a:1022490806093

[19] Kimura R, Murata T. Influence of alkylamides of glutamic acid and related compounds on the central nervous system. I. Central depressant effect of theanine. Chemical & Pharmaceutical Bulletin (Tokyo). 1971;**19**(6):1257-1261. DOI: 10.1248/cpb.19.1257

[20] Heese T, Jenkinson J, Love C, Milam R, Perkins L, Adams C, et al. Anxiolytic effects of L-theanine – a component of green tea - when combined with midazolam, in the male Sprague-Dawley rat. AANA Journal. 2009;**77**(6):445-449

[21] Wakabayashi C, Numakawa T, Ninomiya M, Chiba S, Kunugi H. Behavioral and molecular evidence for psychotropic effects in L-theanine. Psychopharmacology. 2012;**219**(4):1099-1109. DOI: 10.1007/s00213-011-2440-z

[22] Yamada T, Terashima T, Kawano S, Furuno R, Okubo T, Juneja LR, et al. Theanine, gamma-glutamylethylamide, a unique amino acid in tea leaves, modulates neurotransmitter concentrations in the brain striatum interstitium in conscious rats. Amino Acids. 2009;**36**(1):21-27. DOI: 10.1007/s00726-007-0020-7

[23] Liao J, Wu X, Xing Z, Li Q, Duan Y, Fang W, et al. gamma-Aminobutyric Acid (GABA) accumulation in Tea (*Camellia sinensis* L.) through the GABA shunt and polyamine degradation pathways under anoxia. Journal of Agricultural and Food Chemistry. 2017;**65**(14):3013-3018. DOI: 10.1021/acs.jafc.7b00304

[24] Wu QY, Ma SZ, Zhang WW, Yao KB, Chen L, Zhao F, et al. Accumulating pathways of gamma-aminobutyric acid during anaerobic and aerobic sequential incubations in fresh tea leaves. Food Chemistry. 2018;**240**:1081-1086. DOI: 10.1016/j.foodchem.2017.08.004

[25] Alcazar A, Ballesteros O, Jurado JM, Pablos F, Martin MJ, Vilches JL, et al. Differentiation of green, white, black, Oolong, and Pu-erh teas according to

their free amino acids content. Journal of Agricultural and Food Chemistry. 2007;**55**(15):5960-5965. DOI: 10.1021/jf070601a

[26] Ekborg-Ott KH, Taylor A, Armstrong DW. Varietal differences in the total and enantiomeric composition of theanine in tea. Journal of Agricultural and Food Chemistry. 1997;**45**(2):353-363. DOI: 10.1021/jf960432m

[27] Keenan EK, Finnie MDA, Jones PS, Rogers PJ, Priestley CM. How much theanine in a cup of tea? Effects of tea type and method of preparation. Food Chemistry. 2011;**125**(2):588-594. DOI: 10.1016/j.foodchem.2010.08.071

[28] Zuo Y. Simultaneous determination of catechins, caffeine and gallic acids in green, Oolong, black and pu-erh teas using HPLC with a photodiode array detector. Talanta. 2002;**57**(2):307-316. DOI: 10.1016/s0039-9140(02)00030-9

[29] Astill C, Birch MR, Dacombe C, Humphrey PG, Martin PT. Factors affecting the caffeine and polyphenol contents of black and green tea infusions. Journal of Agricultural and Food Chemistry. 2001;**49**(11):5340-5347. DOI: 10.1021/jf010759+

[30] Fernandez PL, Martin MJ, Gonzalez AG, Pablos F. HPLC determination of catechins and caffeine in tea. Differentiation of green, black and instant teas. The Analyst. 2000;**125**(3):421-425. DOI: 10.1039/a909219f

[31] Komes D, Horžić D, Belščak A, Kovačević Ganič K, Baljak A. Determination of caffeine content in tea and Maté tea by using different methods. Czech Journal of Food Science. 2009;**27**(1):S213

[32] Tang GY, Zhao CN, Xu XY, Gan RY, Cao SY, Liu Q, et al. Phytochemical composition and antioxidant capacity of 30 Chinese Teas. Antioxidants. 2019;**8**(6):19. DOI: 10.3390/antiox8060180

[33] Diana M, Quilez J, Rafecas M. γ-Aminobutyric acid as a bioactive compound in foods: A review. Journal of Functional Foods. 2014;**10**:407-420. DOI: 10.1016/j.jff.2014.07.004

[34] Jin YH, Hong JH, Lee J-H, Yoon H, Pawluk AM, Yun SJ, et al. Lactic acid fermented green tea with *Levilactobacillus brevis* capable of producing γ-aminobutyric acid. Fermentation. 2021;**7**(3):20. DOI: 10.3390/fermentation7030110

[35] Jin Y, Tu J, Han X, Zhuo J, Liu G, Han Y, et al. Characteristics of mulberry leaf powder enriched with gamma-aminobutyric acid and its antioxidant capacity as a potential functional food ingredient. Frontiers in Nutrition. 2022;**9**:900718. DOI: 10.3389/fnut.2022.900718

[36] Takayama M, Matsukura C, Ariizumi T, Ezura H. Activating glutamate decarboxylase activity by removing the autoinhibitory domain leads to hyper gamma-aminobutyric acid (GABA) accumulation in tomato fruit. Plant Cell Reports. 2017;**36**(1):103-116. DOI: 10.1007/s00299-016-2061-4

[37] Ezura H. Letter to the Editor: The World's First CRISPR Tomato Launched to a Japanese Market: The Social-Economic Impact of its Implementation on Crop Genome Editing. Plant & Cell Physiology. 2022;**3**. DOI: 10.1093/pcp/pcac048